Taylor's Diagnostic and Therapeutic Challenges

Taylor's Diagnostic and Therapeutic Challenges
A Handbook

Robert B. Taylor, M.D.   Editor
Professor Emeritus
Department of Family Medicine
Oregon Health & Science University
   School of Medicine
Portland, Oregon

Associate Editors

Alan K. David, M.D.
Professor and Chairman
Department of Family and
   Community Medicine
Medical College of Wisconsin
Milwaukee, Wisconsin

Scott A. Fields, M.D.
Professor and Vice Chairman
Department of Family Medicine
Oregon Health & Science University
   School of Medicine
Portland, Oregon

D. Melessa Phillips, M.D.
Professor and Chairman
Department of Family Medicine
University of Mississippi School
   of Medicine
Jackson, Mississippi

Joseph E. Scherger, M.D., M.P.H.
Clinical Professor
Department of Family and
   Preventive Medicine
University of California, San Diego
   School of Medicine
San Diego, California

With 19 Illustrations

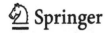 Springer

Robert B. Taylor, M.D.
Professor Emeritus
Department of Family Medicine
Oregon Health & Science University
  School of Medicine
Portland, OR 97201-3098, USA

Associate Editors

Alan K. David, M.D.
Professor and Chairman
Department of Family and
  Community Medicine
Medical College of Wisconsin
Milwaukee, WI 53226-0509, USA

Scott A. Fields, M.D.
Professor and Vice Chairman
Department of Family Medicine
Oregon Health & Science University
  School of Medicine
Portland, OR 97201-3098, USA

D. Melessa Phillips, M.D.
Professor and Chairman
Department of Family Medicine
University of Mississippi School
  of Medicine
Jackson, MS 39216-4500, USA

Joseph E. Scherger, M.D., M.P.H.
Clinical Professor
Department of Family and
  Preventive Medicine
University of California, San Diego
  School of Medicine
San Diego, California 92103-0801

ISBN 0-387-22337-1   Printed on acid-free paper.

Printed in the United States of America.   (MP/MV)

9 8 7 6 5 4 3 2 1   SPIN 10995990

springeronline.com

Taylor's Diagnostic and Therapeutic Challenges
A Handbook

Robert B. Taylor, M.D.   Editor
Professor Emeritus
Department of Family Medicine
Oregon Health & Science University
    School of Medicine
Portland, Oregon

Associate Editors
Alan K. David, M.D.
Professor and Chairman
Department of Family and
    Community Medicine
Medical College of Wisconsin
Milwaukee, Wisconsin

Scott A. Fields, M.D.
Professor and Vice Chairman
Department of Family Medicine
Oregon Health & Science University
    School of Medicine
Portland, Oregon

D. Melessa Phillips, M.D.
Professor and Chairman
Department of Family Medicine
University of Mississippi School
    of Medicine
Jackson, Mississippi

Joseph E. Scherger, M.D., M.P.H.
Clinical Professor
Department of Family and
    Preventive Medicine
University of California, San Diego
    School of Medicine
San Diego, California

With 19 Illustrations

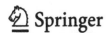 Springer

Robert B. Taylor, M.D.
Professor Emeritus
Department of Family Medicine
Oregon Health & Science University
  School of Medicine
Portland, OR 97201-3098, USA

Associate Editors
Alan K. David, M.D.
Professor and Chairman
Department of Family and
  Community Medicine
Medical College of Wisconsin
Milwaukee, WI 53226-0509, USA

Scott A. Fields, M.D.
Professor and Vice Chairman
Department of Family Medicine
Oregon Health & Science University
  School of Medicine
Portland, OR 97201-3098, USA

D. Melessa Phillips, M.D.
Professor and Chairman
Department of Family Medicine
University of Mississippi School
  of Medicine
Jackson, MS 39216-4500, USA

Joseph E. Scherger, M.D., M.P.H.
Clinical Professor
Department of Family and
  Preventive Medicine
University of California, San Diego
  School of Medicine
San Diego, California 92103-0801

ISBN 0-387-22337-1   Printed on acid-free paper.

Printed in the United States of America.   (MP/MV)

9 8 7 6 5 4 3 2 1   SPIN 10995990

springeronline.com

Preface

This book presents the approach to selected problems that clinicians often find difficult to diagnose or treat. At first, the topics may seem eclectic, but they have been chosen to reflect areas in which I—as a clinician like you—always seem to need to know more (such as genetic disorders and diabetes mellitus), am sometime puzzled as to the etiology (such as headache, thyroid disease, anemia, fatigue, and skin rashes), or am frustrated when problems sometimes do not respond to my best management efforts (such as when patients overeat, drink too much alcohol, or misuse drugs). Also in the latter group are sleep disorders, chronic pain, and other entities discussed in the pages that follow.

In fact, what the seemingly diverse topics presented here share in common is that they all cause both patients and physicians more than their share of challenges.

The chapters in this book are drawn from the sixth edition of the large reference book, *Family Medicine: Principles and Practice,* which is widely used by family physicians in the United States and abroad. The publisher and I believe that, in addition to family physicians, the chapters in this book will also be useful to other clinicians providing primary care, such as general internists, general pediatricians, nurse practitioners, and physician assistants. The price of the "big book" can be a deterrent to some; publication of a smaller book on focused topics allows clinicians to purchase a book on the topics that meet their specific needs. In addition, some find pocket-sized manuals easier to handle than larger, heavy books.

Whatever the reason you picked up this book, I hope that you find it useful in your daily care of patients. Comments are welcome.

Robert B. Taylor, M.D.

Clinical Practice Notice

Everyone involved with the preparation of this book has worked very hard to assure that information presented here is accurate and that it represents accepted clinical practices. These efforts include confirming that drug recommendations and dosages discussed in this text are in accordance with current practice at the time of publication. Nevertheless, therapeutic recommendations and dosage schedules change with reports of ongoing research, changes in government recommendations, reports of adverse drug reactions, and other new information.

A few recommendations and drug uses described herein have Food and Drug Administration (FDA) clearance for limited use in restricted settings. It is the responsibility of the clinician to determine the FDA status of any drug selection, drug dosage, or device recommended to patients.

The reader should check the package insert for each drug to determine any change in indications or dosage as well as for any precautions or warnings. This admonition is especially true when the drug considered is new or infrequently used by the clinician.

The use of the information in this book in a specific clinical setting or situation is the professional responsibility of the clinician. The authors, editors, or publisher are not responsible for errors, omissions, adverse effects, or any consequences arising from the use of information in this book, and make no warranty, expressed or implied, with respect to the completeness, timeliness, or accuracy of the book's contents.

Contents

Contributors

John P. Allen, Ph.D., M.P.A., Chief, Treatment Research Branch, National Institute on Alcohol Abuse and Alcoholism, Rockville, MD

John W. Bachman, M.D., Professor of Medicine, Mayo Medical School; Consultant, Department of Family Medicine, Mayo Clinic, Rochester, MN

Thomas L. Campbell, M.D., Professor, Department of Family Medicine and Department of Psychiatry, University of Rochester School of Medicine and Dentistry, Rochester, NY

Frank S. Celestino, M.D., Associate Professor and Director of Geriatrics, Department of Family and Community Medicine, Wake Forest University School of Medicine, Winston-Salem, NC

Kathy Cole-Kelly, M.S.W., M.S., Associate Professor of Family Medicine, Case Western Reserve University School of Medicine, Cleveland, OH

Gerald M. Cross, M.D., Command Surgeon, United States Army FORSCOM, Atlanta, GA

James J. Deckert, M.D., Associate Clinical Professor of Family and Community Medicine, University of Missouri–Columbia, School of Medicine; Clinical Faculty, Mercy Family Medicine Residency Program and Geriatric Services, St. John's Mercy Medical Center, St. Louis, MO

Enrique S. Fernandez, M.D., M.S.Ed., Family Physician, Miami, FL

Michael B. Harper, M.D., Professor of Family Medicine, Louisiana State University Health Sciences Center, Shreveport, LA

Kenneth A. Hirsch, M.D., Ph.D., Head, Inpatient Mental Health Services, Naval Medical Center, San Diego, CA

Thomas A. Johnson, Jr., M.D., Clinical Professor of Family and Community Medicine, University of Missouri–Columbia School of Medicine; Clinical Faculty, Mercy Family Medicine Residency Program, St. John's Mercy Medical Center, St. Louis, MO

Daniel T. Lee, M.D., Assistant Clinical Professor of Family Medicine, University of California-Los Angeles School of Medicine, Los Angeles; Faculty, Santa Monica-UCLA Medical Center Family Practice Residency Program, Santa Monica, CA

Susan H. McDaniel, Ph.D., Professor, Department of Psychiatry (Psychology) and Department of Family Medicine, University of Rochester School of Medicine and Dentistry, Rochester, NY

Samuel C. Matheny, M.D., M.P.H., Claire Louise Caudill Professor and Chair, Department of Family Practice, University of Kentucky College of Medicine, Lexington, KY

E.J. Mayeaux, Jr., M.D., Associate Professor of Family Medicine, Louisiana State University Health Sciences Center, Shreveport, LA

Carole Nistler, M.D., Private Practice, Olmsted Community Hospital, Rochester, MN

Michael T. Railey, M.D., Assistant Professor of Community and Family Medicine, St. Louis University School of Medicine; Forest Park Hospital Family Medicine Residency Program, St. Louis, MO

John Saultz, M.D., Professor and Chairman, Department of Family Medicine, Oregon Health & Science University School of Medicine, Portland, OR

Jerome E. Schulz, M.D., Clinical Professor of Family Medicine, East Carolina University Brody School of Medicine; Pitt County Memorial Hospital, Greenville, NC

John P. Sheehan, M.D., Associate Clinical Professor of Medicine, Case Western Reserve University School of Medicine, Cleveland, OH

Charles Kent Smith, M.D., Dorothy Jones Weatherhead Professor of Family Medicine, Case Western Reserve University School of Medicine, Cleveland, OH

Jeannette E. South-Paul, M.D., Professor and Chair, Department of Family Medicine and Clinical Epidemiology, University of Pittsburgh School of Medicine, Pittsburgh, PA

Angela W. Tang, M.D., Assistant Professor of Medicine, University of California–Los Angeles School of Medicine, Los Angeles; Department of Medical Education, Saint Mary Medical Center, Internal Medicine Residency, Long Beach, CA

Margaret M. Ulchaker, M.S.N., R.N., C.D.E., NP-C., Clinical Instructor, Frances Payne Bolton School of Nursing, Case Western Reserve University, Cleveland, OH

Daniel J. Van Durme, M.D., Associate Professor and Vice-Chairman, Department of Family Medicine, University of South Florida College of Medicine, Tampa, FL

Thomas J. Zuber, M.D., Associate Physician, Department of Family Medicine and Preventive Medicine, Emory University School of Medicine, Atlanta, GA

1
Cultural, Race, and Ethnicity Issues in Health Care

Enrique S. Fernandez,
Jeannette E. South-Paul,
and Samuel C. Matheny

The world is facing movements of peoples unparalleled in history. Even the heartland of the American continent, which has seen few new population groups since the European immigration of the 19th century, has felt the effects of this restive population shift during the late 1980s and 1990s. Physicians who themselves have had little experience outside their own cultural environment are now dealing with health and social issues of patients who approach their surroundings in profoundly different ways than they might themselves. Yet the differences have always been present.

Cultural groups exist in the United States in many forms, and each has the potential for its members to interpret their world in a different manner. In fact, the subtlety of the differences between peoples with common languages and outward appearances may cause even more misunderstandings and concerns than those with more obvious external dissimilarities.

Western Medicine in the Context of Race, Ethnicity, and Culture

The concepts of race, ethnicity, and culture frequently are addressed interchangeably. Racial distinctions are probably the ones most commonly made in clinical settings—often as part of a rote introductory clause in a patient history—and often have limited clinical utility, occasionally establishing misleading and potentially harmful patient stereotypes. An appreciation of how ethnic and cultural factors influence patient health and the clinical encounter is an important consideration when providing effective disease prevention, health promotion, and treatment interventions.

Race

Racial classifications are generally defined by physical characteristics (e.g., skin color, facial features, hair type) that are shared by a group of people. They form the basis for an assumption of a shared genetic heritage among groups of humans. A presumption of shared genetic traits by a group of people who bear superficial similarity might apply to inbred populations that are geographically isolated, but this distinction becomes less meaningful when one considers the intermingling of human populations over the centuries. When one considers that there is more genetic variation to be found within a given race than between two different races, ascribing genetic traits based on race designations alone adds little to the medical decision-making process.[1]

Ethnicity

The word *ethnic* is defined by the *American Heritage Dictionary* as, "of, or relating to, sizable groups of people sharing a common and distinctive racial, national, religious, linguistic, or cultural heritage." Derivations can also be linked with race. The word *ethnicity* is derived from the Greek terms *ethnos*, referring to the people of a nation or a tribe, and *ethnikos*, equating with "national" or "nationality."[2] Ethnicity thus refers to a group affiliation, which is normally expressed in terms of cultural characteristics. Although cultural characteristics are associated with ethnic groups, the members of such groups define and transmit cultural norms.

Culture

Culture can be described as the knowledge, skills, and attitudes learned and passed on from one generation to the next. Cultural identity is a dynamic, lifelong process that is constantly molded and refined by personal experience. Cultural identity thus incorporates a fluidity that defies conclusive statements about the characteristics of populations that share a common culture. Cultural norms can be modified by level of education, socioeconomic status, and the number of generations an individual is removed from the initial migration of his or her family from one society to another. Indeed, there are often more similarities to be found between two individuals of the same socioeconomic status who are from different cultures than between two individuals of the same culture who differ in socioeconomic status.[3] The degree of cultural identity determines the role that family plays for the individual, as well as communication patterns, affective styles, and personal values regarding level of control, individualism, collectivism, spirituality, and religious beliefs. Culture is also modified by age, sex, vocation, disability, and sexual orientation.

Health professionals often participate in a variety of cultures simultaneously: the culture of a family of origin, that of the family of a significant other, the profession entered, or even occasionally a culture dictated by other factors, such as sexual orientation. In turn, the patient presents with a variety of layers of the same cultural cake; recognizing these influences can be a complex, subtle, profound task. As physicians, it is useful to consider the origins of our medical model and how that model determines our approach to patients.

Western Medical Model

The Western medical model was developed in contemporary Western society as a powerful analytic tool to deal with illness. This model developed around the classical Greek myth of Pandora's box in which disease is an intrusion superimposed on humans from the outside. The concept defines the social system within which a defined professional group (i.e., physicians) takes responsibility for the care of persons with compromised function. The model determines the type of questions raised during the history-taking process. Emphasis on physical symptoms often predisposes the interviewer to neglect material of potentially great value (e.g., the social system of the patient). Indeed, cultural factors may create profound differences between patient and physician perceptions of health.

In our medical model, disease is defined as some form of abnormal structure or bodily function that leads to a specific pathology. In this context, disease is a condition most readily identified by the health professional, who attempts to place it in terms of the classification of disorders that has traditionally developed in Western medicine.

Illness, on the other hand, pertains more to the individual's feelings of a negative state of being or social function; it is the human experience of sickness. Illness then may be said to be the perception of the patient, whereas disease is the perception of the health provider. In many cases these two views of sickness coincide, but frequently there are major discrepancies between them. For example, a physician may detect an elevated blood pressure and communicate the diagnosis of hypertension to a patient, who feels perfectly well and has no symptoms but may feel ill only when beginning the antihypertensive medication. Conversely, a Mexican patient may decide that he or she is suffering from *susto*, or emotional fright. This description of a state of anxiety may fail to be identified by a physician but would be completely accepted and understood by anyone in this person's cultural group. Illness for the patient may have several distinct meanings. It may represent a threat to the individual, in that it may be perceived as possible punishment for a wrongdoing. Many cultures, including groups in the United States, have on occasion viewed various epidemics in this fashion, including human immunodeficiency virus (HIV) infection.

Illness may be also viewed as a loss, as with the loss of independence or the ability to communicate effectively, as would occur following a cerebrovascular accident or with other chronic, debilitating conditions. Conversely, illness may be viewed as a gain, in that there may be advantages to being ill that are more acceptable to society.

Clark[4] described, in her classic study of a Mexican-American community, a pregnant woman who had been struck by her husband. She sought the aid of a *curandera* to prevent a case of *susto* in her unborn child, as described above. This socially acceptable action allowed her to gain community sympathy against her husband for the physical abuse, which would otherwise have been denied her. The husband was convinced of the error of his ways, and the couple was reunited.[4]

Lastly, the illness may convey no particular significance to the individual patient and may be viewed as a normal part of life. Because biomedicine has been largely interested in the treatment of disease, little attention has been paid to interpreting the meaning of illness. Kleinman et al[5] noted that "because illness experience is an intimate part of social systems of meanings and rules for behavior, it is strongly influenced by culture." The lack of attention to illness, and therefore to culture, often results in noncompliance or dissatisfaction with health care delivery.

Population Demographic Shifts

Today minority populations—those who often do not subscribe to the Western biomedical model—are the fastest growing segments of the United States population, representing a substantial proportion of the work force for the 21st century.[6] Southeast Asians and Central Americans made up the largest numbers of immigrants in the late 1970s and 1980s. Census 2000 data revealed dramatic changes from what was initially projected from 1990 results. For the first time, non-Hispanic whites make up less than 70% of the overall population. African Americans and Hispanics each comprise 12% of the population, although Hispanics grew by 61% from numbers in 1990.[7] Asian Americans grew by more than 45% to make up 3.6% of the current population, while American-Indian representation remains low at 0.7%. Furthermore, the 2000 census allowed a change in options for self-identification. Subsequently, 6.8 million people identified themselves as multiracial.[8] Physicians of the 21st century will provide care to a population whose characteristics differ markedly from the population in the United States today. Over the next 30 years, the U.S. population will be larger by almost one third, it will be more diverse, and it will be older. The U.S. Census Bureau estimates that by the year 2050 only 52% of the American population will be white, 16% black, 22% Latino/Hispanic, and 10% Asian. These projected demographic trends will influence significantly the patterns of disease and the health care of the population.[9]

Morbidity and Mortality Variations

The health care system is a reflection of current American society. Lack of access to health care due to an inability to pay or lack of insurance, absence of translators when English is not the patient's language, differing health practices, psychosocial and environmental factors, and cultural differences are all major contributors to differences in health status among the various subgroups that comprise the American population.

Health Status of African Americans

A persistent gap exists in the United States between the health status of African Americans and that of white Americans. Infant mortality for African Americans continues to exceed that of whites and is merely a prelude to other negative health indicators through life: Being black is now considered a health hazard.[10] Even when income differences are factored in and financial access to prenatal care is ensured, African-American women use prenatal care later and less intensively.[11,12]

In 1990 the life expectancy at birth for African-American boys and girls was 64.5 and 73.6 years, respectively, whereas that for white boys and girls was 72.7 and 79.4 years, respectively. The infant mortality rate (per 1,000 births) in 1993 was 6.8 for whites compared with 16.5 for African Americans. There was a larger decline in mortality for African- American infants from 1992 to 1993 than for white infants, but the dramatic differences persist.[13]

Health Status of Hispanics

Hispanics are at increased risk for diabetes, hypertension, tuberculosis, HIV infection, alcoholism, cirrhosis, specific cancers, and violent deaths. Poverty and lack of health insurance are the greatest impediments to health care for Hispanics. One third to one fifth of various Hispanic populations (and one fifth of the African-American non-Hispanic population) are uninsured for medical expenses, compared with one tenth of the white non-Hispanic population.

Health Status of Native Americans

Native Americans suffer some of the worst health in the nation and the lowest social status even among minorities and underserved people. Access to health care for Native Americans is more difficult than for the rest of the U.S. population because of their geographic isolation in villages and communities that are large in area and have large reservations, poor transportation, lack of efficient communications systems, and lack of running water and sewage disposal. Travel may require long distances on dirt roads or by air. Native Americans are younger, less educated, less likely to be employed, and poorer than the general population. These factors, combined with high rates of sexually transmitted disease and drug use, favor the spread of HIV. Alcoholism exacts a terrible toll among many Native Americans. Tribal, cultural, educational, economic, and geographic diversity exist among Native Americans and affect their health care.[14]

Health Status of Asian-Pacific Americans

Important ethnic differences in risk factors indicate that Asian-Pacific American (APA) groups should be targeted for public health efforts concerned with obesity, hypertension, hypercholesterolemia, and smoking.[14] Conditions endemic in the country of origin and case rates for tuberculosis among APAs (44.5/100,000) are greater than for other minority groups: African Americans (29.1/100,000), Hispanics (20.6/100,000), and American Indians/Alaska Natives (14.6/100,000).[14]

Recognizing Cultural Differences

How we interpret and deal with illness is based on our explanations of illness—explanations that are specific to the social positions we occupy and the belief system we employ. These factors have been shown to modify how we perceive symptoms, what labels we attach to particular illnesses, and how we interpret these labels. How we communicate our health problems, the manner in which we present our symptoms, when and from whom we seek care, how long we remain in care, and our evaluation of that care are affected by cultural beliefs.[15]

Most health care providers have a collection of anecdotes about noncompliance by ethnically different patients. As these issues have been studied by medical sociologists and anthropologists, the focus of the problem has come to rest on the provider as much as on the patient. The "fallacy of the empty vessel" is a phrase coined by anthropologists to describe cross-cultural blindness. People tend to ignore parts of cultures (e.g., religion, health care traditions) that differ from their own. The anthropologist Hazel Weidman noted that orthodox health care providers often view Western health institutions as introducing something of significance into ethnic communities where nothing existed before. Thus the existing health traditions in such communities are ignored.

Borkan and Neher[16] developed a framework for use in family practice training programs, modeled after one developed by Bennett.[17] Bennett suggested a model with stages of individual development relative to cultural sensitivity. The Borkan and Neher model built on this model by recognizing the importance of ethnosensitivity to understanding the whole person and by advancing doctor–patient communication. They recognized that the individual trainee's relationship with other cultures may be more complex than implied by Bennett's model. The level of sensitivity exhibited by a trainee can vary according to the group encountered (e.g., sensitive and empathetic to Southeast Asians and culturally unaware with respect to Haitians).

Thus Borkan and Neher suggested a model of ethnosensitivity consisting of seven stages, with curricular strategies and goals to address each stage: (1) fear, (2) denial, (3) superiority, (4) minimization, (5) relativism, (6) empathy, and (7) integration. Fear is the most problematic stage because it may preclude any efforts to provide medical care. Denial can be addressed by attempting to heighten the awareness of trainees to cultural differences. Superiority is the stage where differences are recognized, but trainees tend to rank them according to their own value system. With minimization, cultural differences are viewed as unimportant against the background of basic human similarities. Ethnic and cultural differences are finally acknowledged in the relativism stage and are no longer seen as threatening. With empathy, the trainee can adopt the frame of reference of patients in order to experience events as they would. Integration is the most advanced level of physician awareness and allows the practitioner to become enmeshed in more than one culture.

Physicians and patients have their own cultural identities. Only by recognizing where one is on the cultural continuum can each encounter be placed in perspective. Knowing oneself and one's views and assumptions, therefore, is the first step in assessing and understanding others.

Individuals often submerge their identification with their past cultural traditions and adopt the traditions of their new country. Harwood[18] enumerated five major factors that may contribute to variation in an individual subscribing to the standards of a group of origin: (1) acculturation, (2) level of income, (3) occupation, (4) area of origin in the mother country, and (5) religion. The level of acculturation may be the most difficult to ascertain by a clinician; eight screening points are delineated for detecting those individuals who tend to be most acculturated into middle-class American standards:

1. Relatively high level of formal education
2. Greater generational removal from immigrant status
3. Low level of involvement within an ethnic or family social network
4. Experience with medical services that incorporates patient education and personal care
5. Previous experience with particular diseases in the immediate family
6. Immigration to this country at an early age
7. Urban, as opposed to rural, origin
8. Limited migration back and forth to the mother country

Harwood pointed out, however, that in times of stress, all individuals may revert to beliefs they do not consistently hold at other times.

Crucial Factors in the Cross-Cultural Clinical Encounter

It should be the goal of any clinical encounter that both the patient and the clinician are able to develop mutual understanding and feel comfortable in the relationship, and that quality health care is delivered in an efficient and timely manner beneficial to the patient. Several factors are necessary for successful physician–patient experience: an awareness of certain core cultural issues, an understanding of the meaning of illness to the patient, an ability for the physician to negotiate across this "cultural divide," and clarity of communication. Certain elements have been identified as essential for assessing the cultural attributes of a person, community, or group of people and have been termed the domains of culture.

Language

Word usage may not be the same in the cultures of the clinician and the patient, and care should be taken to use simple words that can be easily understood in communication. If a patient does not speak the language of the clinician or vice versa, it is especially important to attempt to alleviate areas of confusion. Up to one third of minority and immigrant households in the United States may be described as linguistically isolated. These are households where no one over the age of 14 speaks English. This poses significant challenges for the physician–patient encounter, especially when translators are not readily available.

A physician, newly arrived at his post on an Indian reservation in the southwestern United States, paid a courtesy call on the chair of the Tribal Council for the group with whom he was assigned. During the course of a half-hour of pleasant conversation, the chair told him that he hoped he would enjoy his stay and find the reservation pleasant. The physician answered by saying that he was sure that he would enjoy his tenure, but that his primary purpose here was to practice medicine and that his enjoyment of his setting was of secondary importance. Within a few hours, word had gotten out on the reservation that the physician had come to the reservation to "practice" (that is, experiment) on the tribe, a misunderstanding that nearly caused his transfer.

Time

Different cultures may hold different concepts of time, which can provide several areas of misunderstanding. For patients from certain cultures, being on time for an appointment may mean within a 15-minute window, within an hour, or within a half-day. The concept of future time may also vary. In some rural-based cultures, advising patients that they must undertake certain preventive measures to prevent illness at some future time may be difficult to fathom, as their consideration of time may exist only in the present or the next season.

Decision Makers

In some cultures, important decisions, including those involving medical care, may be a communal decision by the extended family or by a designated family leader instead of the spouse or other nuclear family members. In an attempt to expedite an important decision, physicians may alienate these designated decision makers or the patient. Conversely, when the family leader is the patient, other family members may be reticent to accept responsibility for decision making in the event of the incapacity of the family leader involved.

Illness Models

There may be significant differences of opinion between the clinician and the patient, and not just concerning the etiology of certain symptoms. The very recognition of certain conditions as "illness" by the patient and the physician may vary.

An African-American patient presented to a major city hospital emergency room, complaining of nervousness, "shakes," and weight loss over the past several months. He had been unable to sleep and expressed generalized anxiety. Upon more intensive questioning, it was determined by one of the nurses that he felt that one of his former female companions had placed a curse on him, known in the southern coastal region as "the root."

It was difficult in this case for the clinician to accept both the patient's explanation of the etiology of the symptoms and the very existence of the illness described.

Treatment and Effectiveness of Intercession

On occasion, the patient and clinician agree that significant illness is present, but the reasons for the illness and the appropriate treatment may differ significantly.

A woman who had recently moved to Los Angeles from central Mexico presented an 11-month-old child to a physician's office with signs of diarrhea and mild dehydration. The mother, through an interpreter, told the clinician that the child had *mollera caida*, literally "fallen fontanelle." Her method of treatment was to place salt on the fontanelle, turn the child upside down to fill out the sunken spots, and give the child *manzanilla* (chamomile) tea. The clinician, on the other hand, was concerned about the diarrheal etiology and wished to initiate oral rehydration.

Traditional Role of Healer

For better or worse, much of the outcome deriving from the encounter between the clinician and patient depends on the expectations and experiences of the patient in his or her cultural group. If the healer is expected to be omnipotent and make the diagnosis by observation only, questioning by the clinician may be taken as a sign of ignorance or incompetence. The healer may also have been an integral part of the community of the individual and be well respected and liked, or the converse may have been true. These attitudes may be transferred over to the clinician, who is unaware of the expectations bestowed by the patient.

Managing Cross-Cultural Differences

Cultural sensitivity training is implemented regularly in only a small number of medical schools. A 1991 study revealed that only 13% of schools offered cultural sensitivity courses to their students, with all but one being optional.[19] A national survey of family practice residencies in 1985 revealed that only 26% provided learning experiences in culturally sensitive health care.[20] However, a 1998 Association of American Medical Colleges' survey revealed that almost 70% of the 94 schools that responded taught courses in cultural competence. Fifteen percent plan to introduce it into the curriculum in the near future. Approximately one third (36%) of residencies offer some kind of formal teaching in this area.[21,22] The Liaison Committee on Medical Education also launched a new Diversity Standard in May 1999. It notes that students must understand and be able to deal with various belief systems, cultural biases, and other culturally determined factors that influence the manner in which different people experience illness and respond to advice and treatment. Furthermore, the Society of Teachers of Family Medicine (STFM) Task Force on Cross-Cultural Experiences published recommended curriculum guidelines to assist in training family physicians to provide culturally sensitive and competent health care.[23] The goal in such training is competence in recognizing bias, prejudice, and discrimination, using cultural resources, and overcoming cultural barriers to enhance primary care.

Cultural differences can easily lead to differences in the models by which a clinician or a patient might explain a presenting condition and the most effective course of management. Figure 1.1 suggests the ultimate goal in cross-cultural medicine: effective integration of patient and clinician knowledge to produce a shared model

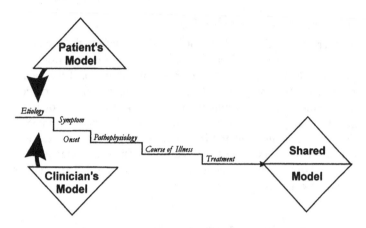

Fig. 1.1. Integration of patient and clinician knowledge to produce a shared model of care.

of care. When a clinician recognizes that a possibility exists for significant differences in the explanatory models of illness and the approach for management, it is necessary to supplement the traditional history to ascertain these issues and develop a plan for coming to some understanding with the patient.

LEARN Model

Berlin and Fowkes[24] developed an instrument useful to clinicians for negotiating the differences that may exist between patient and provider. The LEARN acronym is based on the following five steps (Fig. 1.2).

1. Listen. Ask the patient such questions as "What do you think is causing this problem?" "Why do you think it started in this way?" "What do you think this illness is doing to you?" "What do you fear the most about this illness?" "How severe is it?" "What do you think is going to happen to you?" "What kind of treatment do you think you should receive?" These questions give the clinician the framework to understand the patient's model of etiology of illness and the opportunity to demonstrate empathy and understanding.

2. Explain. With this step the clinician explains his or her interpretation of the medical condition. It may be nothing more than a supposition, but it is important that the clinician present an understanding based on Western medical tradition.

LISTEN WITH SYMPATHY & UNDERSTANDING TO
THE PATIENT'S PERCEPTION OF THE PROBLEM

EXPLAIN YOUR PERCEPTIONS OF THE PROBLEM

ACKNOWLEDGE AND DISCUSS DIFFERENCES &
SIMILARITIES

RECOMMEND TREATMENT

NEGOTIATE TREATMENT

Fig. 1.2. Managing cross-cultural differences: the LEARN model. (*Source:* Berlin and Fowkes,[24] with permission.)

3. Acknowledge. It is important to acknowledge the patient's explanatory model and begin to develop areas where agreement can be met and conflicts between explanatory models can be resolved.
4. Recommend. In this stage, the clinician can recommend a plan for action that incorporates the patient's explanatory models of illness and those of the clinician.
5. Negotiate. Berlin and Fowkes consider this step the most important. It includes incorporating the patient's and clinician's understanding and plans. The final step may well be an amalgamation of the two belief systems that can be mutually tolerated.

In the case of the child with the *mollera caida*, the physician listened carefully to the mother's explanation of the cause of the sunken fontanelle. She then explained to the mother that in her view the cause of the sunken fontanelle was the diarrhea, but acknowledged the concern of the mother for restoring the fullness of the fontanelle. Because the mother was using boiled *manzanilla* tea, she negotiated with the mother to add sufficient nutrients to the tea to compose an oral rehydration solution and encouraged this part of the traditional treatment to continue.

Working with Translators

Special care is needed with interviews involving translators to ensure the accuracy and completeness of the information and the cooperation of the patient. Clinicians must view the translator as part of a team whose members collaborate to arrive at a competent plan for the patient:

1. Look at the patient when speaking. Always address the patient, not the interpreter, and speak in the first person directly to the patient, asking the interpreter to interpret in a direct fashion.
2. Use comforting body language, recognizing that it is instantaneously interpreted by the patient.
3. Whenever possible, explain to the interpreter in advance what you are trying to say and accomplish during the interview.
4. Assume that there will be misunderstandings, particularly when you are using nonprofessional interpreters.
5. Remain aware and test your patient's understanding. Some patients may understand your language even if they choose to use an interpreter; or, conversely, patients who speak fairly well in the language of the clinician may not have the same level of comprehension.
6. Keep the sentence structure simple, avoiding complex phrases.
7. If there are a significant number of patients in your practice who speak a particular language, it alleviates some misunderstanding if the clinician learns as much of the language as possible. This effort increases the trust of the patient and allows the clinician to more readily pick up errors by the interpreter.[25]
8. Be especially wary of the accuracy of interpretation from family members, particularly concerning the sexual or gynecologic history of female patients. In certain cultures it is taboo to discuss these topics with the patient, even when interpreting for the clinician. Also, in many cultures children are particularly problematic when acting as translators.

References

1. Cooper R, David R. The biological concept of race and its application to public health and epidemiology. J Health Polit Policy Law 1986;2:97–116.
2. Betancourt H, Lopez SR. The study of culture, ethnicity, and race in American psychology. Am Psychol 1993;48:629–37.
3. Greenbaum S. Race, ethnicity and culture. San Francisco: USF Center for Teaching Enhancement, 1992.
4. Clark M. Health in the Mexican American culture. Berkeley: University of California Press, 1959.
5. Kleinman A, Eisenberg L, Good B. Culture, illness, and care: clinical lessons from anthropologic and cross-cultural research. Ann Intern Med 1978;88:251–8.

6. Kehrer BH, Burroughs HC. More minorities in health. Menlo Park, CA: Kaiser Forums, 1994.
7. U.S. Bureau of the Census. Population change and distribution 1990 to 2000. Washington, DC: U.S. Census Brief, April 2001.
8. U.S. Bureau of the Census. Overview of race and hispanic origin, Washington, DC: U.S. Census Brief, March 2001.
9. Kehrer BH, Burroughs HC. More minorities in health. Menlo Park, CA: 1994.
10. Gates-Williams J, Jackson MN, Jenkins-Monroe V, Williams LR. The business of preventing African-American infant mortality [special issue]. West J Med 1992;157:350–6.
11. Murray JL, Bernfield M. The differential effect of prenatal care on the incidence of low birthweight among blacks and whites in a prepaid health plan. N Engl J Med 1988;319: 1385–91.
12. Kugler JP, Connell FA, Henley CE. Lack of difference in neonatal mortality between blacks and whites served by the same medical care system. J Fam Pract 1990;30(3):281–7.
13. Rosenberg HM, Ventura SJ, Maurer JD, Hauser RL, Freedman MA. Births and deaths. United States, 1995. Monthly Vital Statistics Rep 1996;45(3)S(2).
14. Lin-Fu JS. Asian and Pacific islander Americans: an overview of demographic characteristics and health issues. Asian Pac Islander J Health 1994;2:20–36.
15. Kleinman A, Eisenberg L, Good B. Culture, illness, and care: clinical lessons from anthropologic and cross-cultural research. Ann Intern Med 1978;88:251–8.
16. Borkan JM, Neher JO. A developmental model of ethnosensitivity in family practice training. Fam Med 1991;23:212–17.
17. Bennett MJ. A developmental approach to training for intercultural sensitivity. Int J Intercultural Rel 1986;10:179–96.
18. Harwood A. Ethnicity and medical care. Boston: Harvard University Press, 1981.
19. Lum CK, Korenman SG. Cultural-sensitivity training in U.S. medical schools. Acad Med 1994;69:239–41.
20. McConarty PC, Farr F. Culture as content in family practice residencies. Presented at the Society of Teachers of Family Medicine 19th Annual Spring Conference, San Diego, May 1986.
21. Personal communication: teaching cultural competence: Danoff D, Asst VP for Medical Education, Washington, DC: AAMC.
22. Greene J. AM News 1999(25 Oct);8–9.
23. Like RC, Steiner P, Rubel AJ. Recommended core curriculum guidelines on culturally sensitive and competent health care. Fam Med 1996;27:291–7.
24. Berlin E, Fowkes WC Jr. A teaching framework for cross-cultural health care—application in family practice. West J Med 1983;934–8.
25. Freebairn J, Gwinup K. Cultural diversity and nursing practice. Irvine, CA: Concept Media, 1979.

2

Family Issues in Health Care

*Thomas L. Campbell,
Susan H. McDaniel, and
Kathy Cole-Kelly*

Caring for families is one of the defining characteristics of family practice. Families are the primary context within which most health problems and illnesses occur and have a powerful influence on health.[1] Most health beliefs and behaviors (e.g., smoking, diet, exercise) are developed and maintained within the family.[2] Marital and family relationships have as powerful an impact on health outcomes as biologic factors,[3] and family interventions have been shown to improve health outcomes for a variety of health problems.[4]

Family members, not health professionals, provide most of the health care for patients. Outside the hospital, health care professionals give advice and suggestions for the acute and chronic illness, but the actual care is usually provided by the patient (self-care) and family members. Chronic illness requires families to adapt and change roles to provide needed care. The aging of the population and increasing medical technology leads to a significant increase in the prevalence of chronic illness and disability and a rise in family caregiving.

Unfortunately, families are often neglected in health care. Our culture is individually oriented, valuing autonomy over connectedness. The impact of serious illness on other family members is often ignored. Family practice developed around the concept of caring for the entire family, yet many family physicians have received inadequate training in how to work with families. Some have even argued that it is not practical and takes too much time to work with families. The ability to work effectively and efficiently with families and to use them as a resource in patient care is an essential skill for all family physicians.

Despite rapid societal changes in the structure and function of families, the family remains the most important relational unit and provides individuals with their most basic needs for physical and emotional safety, health, and well-being. The family can be defined as "any group of people related either biologically, emotionally, or legally."[5] This includes all forms of traditional and nontraditional families, such as unmarried couples, blended families, and gay and lesbian couples. The relevant family context may include family members who live a distance from the patient or all the residents of a community home for the developmentally delayed persons. In daily practice, family physicians are most often involved with family members who live in the same household.

Premises of a Family Systems Approach

There are three basic premises upon which a family systems approach is based. These premises are derived from systems theory, are supported by research, and help guide the clinical application of family systems.

1. A family systems approach is based on a biopsychosocial model of health care in which there is an interrelationship between biologic, psychological, and social processes. This approach places the patient and the illness in a larger framework involving multiple systems. The family-oriented physician must recognize and address the psychosocial factors as well as the biomedical factors in understanding patients and their illness. A systems approach emphasizes the interaction among the different levels of the larger systems and the importance of continuous and reciprocal feedback.
2. The family has an influence on physical and psychological health and well-being. This principle is well supported by research and has important implications for clinical practice. Clinicians must understand how the family can positively and negatively influence health and utilize the information to improve health care. There are several corollaries to this basic premise.
   a. The family is a primary source of many health beliefs and behaviors.

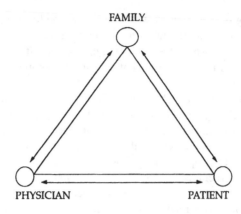

Fig. 2.1. Therapeutic triangle. (*Source:* Doherty and Baird.[6])

    b. The family is an important source of stress and social support.
    c. Physical symptoms may have an adaptive function within a family and be maintained by family patterns.
3. The family is the primary social context in which health care issues are addressed. Although the patient is the primary focus of medical care, the family is often the most important social context that must be understood and considered when delivering health care. It is not useful to think of the family as the "unit of care." Family physicians treat individuals within families, not families themselves. They must consider the family context and address family relationships when they influence health problems. This is important whether a physician cares for only one or every member of a family.

Doherty and Baird[6] have challenged the "illusion of the medical dyad" between the physician and patient and have described the relationship of the physician, patient, and family as a therapeutic triangle (Fig. 2.1). This triangle emphasizes that the family plays a role in all patient encounters regardless of whether family members are present and the need to be cognizant of both the patient–family relationship and the physician–family relationship.

Research on Families and Health

A large body of research has demonstrated the powerful influence that families have on health. There are many randomized controlled trials demonstrating the effectiveness of family interventions for medical disorders.[4] A recent Institute of Medicine report on families, health, and behavior reviewed the research on the influence of family relationships on the management and outcomes of chronic diseases.[7] Several general conclusions can be made from a review of this research:

1. Families have a powerful influence on health and illness. Numerous large epidemiologic studies have demonstrated that social support, particularly from the family, is health promoting. In an 1988 article in the journal *Science*, sociologist James House et al[3] reviewed this research and concluded, "The evidence regarding social relationships and health increasingly approximates the evidence in the 1964 Surgeon General's report that established cigarette smoking as a cause or risk factor for mortality and morbidity from a range of disease. The age-adjusted relative risk ratios are stronger than the relative risks for all cause mortality reported for cigarette smoking."

   Family support affects the outcome of most chronic medical illnesses. After suffering a myocardial infarction (MI), women with few or no family supports have two to three times the mortality rate compared to other women who are recovering from an MI.[8] Many stresses within the family, such as loss of a spouse and divorce, significantly impact morbidity and mortality.

2. Emotional support is the most important and influential type of family support. Social and family support can be divided into different types: instrumental, informational, and emotional. Instrumental support is the actual provision of services (e.g., driving the patient to the hospital) or caregiving (e.g., giving insulin injections) provided by family members. Informational support usually involves giving health-related information, such as advice on whether to seek medical care. Emotional support provides a listening ear, empathy, and the sense that one is cared about and loved. Although there is overlap among these categories, studies suggests that family emotional support has the most important influence on health outcomes and therefore cannot be replaced with social agencies or services that provide instrumental and informational support.

3. Marriage is the most influential family relationship on health. Even after controlling for other factors, marital status affects overall mortality, mortality from specific illnesses, especially cancer and heart disease, and morbidity. Married individuals are healthier than widowed, who are in turn healthier than either divorced

or never-married individuals. Those who are married have healthier lifestyles and less disability, and they live longer. Bereavement or death of a spouse increases mortality, especially for men.[9] Separation and divorce is also associated with increased morbidity and mortality. Studies in psychoimmunology have shown that divorced and unhappily married men and women have poorer immune function than those in healthier marriages.[10]

4. Negative, critical, or hostile family relationships have a stronger influence on health than positive or supportive relationships. In terms of health, "being nasty" is worse than simply not being nice. Research in the mental health field with schizophrenia and depression first demonstrated that family criticism was strongly predictive of relapse and poor outcome.[11,12] Similar results have been found with smoking cessation,[13] weight management,[14] diabetes,[15] asthma, and migraine headaches. Physiologic studies have shown that conflict and criticism between family members can have negative influences on blood pressure,[16] diabetes control,[17] and immune function.

5. Family psychoeducation is an effective intervention for health problems. There is a wide range of types of family interventions that have been used for health problems, from simply providing family members with information about the disease to in-depth family therapy. The most consistently effective and studied family intervention seems to be family psychoeducation, in which family members are given training on how to manage and cope with the illness and provided with emotional and instrumental support.[18]

An excellent example of an effective, family psychoeducational intervention has been developed for family caregivers of Alzheimer disease (AD) patients.[19] In a randomized controlled trial, families attended individual and group instructional and problem-solving sessions where they learned how to manage many of the troublesome behaviors of patients with AD. They also participated in ongoing family support group and can access a crisis intervention service to help them with urgent problems. The caregivers who received this intervention were less depressed and physically healthier than those who did not, and AD patients were able to remain at home for almost a year longer than caregivers in the control group. The savings in nursing home costs were several times the cost of the interventions. This study should serve as a model for other family intervention programs.

This research establishes that families have a strong influence on overall health and on the outcome of specific illnesses. The impact is the greatest for illnesses in which there is a high burden on family caregivers. Effective family interventions range from complex, multifaceted programs (e.g., for AD patients) to educating family members about the illness (e.g., hypertension). To implement any of the interventions, family physicians must know how to work with families and use them as a resource in patient care.

Working with Families

Much of what has been written about working with families has focused on the family conference, the most formal and uncommon form of a family interview. It is useful to distinguish three approaches to working with families: the family-oriented approach with an individual patient, involving family members during a routine office visit, and the family conference or meeting (Table 2.1). In all of these contexts, medical care is enhanced by obtaining information about the family, assessing family relationships, and encouraging appropriate family involvement.

A Family-Oriented Approach with an Individual Patient

A family orientation has more to do with how one thinks about the patient than how many people are in the exam room. Since family physicians meet with individual patients more often than with family members, having a family-oriented approach to all patients is an important skill. This approach complements a patient-centered approach in which the physician explores the patient's experience of illness, an experience that occurs in a family or relational context. The patient's presenting complaint can be thought of as an entrance or window into understanding the patient in the context of the family. By exploring the patient's symptoms and illness, the physician can learn more about the patient's family, its relationship to the presenting complaint, and how the family can be used as resource in treatment. A key to being family oriented is choosing appropriate questions to learn about the psychosocial and family-related issues without the patient feeling that the physician is intruding or suggesting that the problem is "all in your head."

In a qualitative study of exemplar family physicians, Cole-Kelly and colleagues[20] examined the core components of a family-oriented approach with individual patients. These family physicians used both global family questions, such as "How's everyone doing at home?" as well as focused family-oriented questions, such as "How is your

Table 2.1. **Working with Families**

	Family-oriented approach with individual patient	Involving family members in routine office visits	Family conference
Common medical situations	Acute medical problems Self-limiting problems	Well-child and prenatal care Diagnosis of a chronic illness Noncompliance Somatization	Hospitalization Terminal illness Institutionalization Serious family problem/conflict
Percent of time used by physician	60–75%	25–40%	2–5%
Length of visit	10–15 minutes	15–20 minutes	30–40 minutes
How scheduled	Routine care	May need to request family member attendance	Special scheduling and planning

Source: Adapted from McDaniel et al.[5]

wife doing with that new treatment?" The exemplars frequently inquired about other family members and were able to keep a storehouse of family details in their minds that they frequently interspersed in the visits. The physician would commonly punctuate the end of the visit with a greeting to another family member: "Be sure to tell John I said hello."

A risk of being family-oriented with an individual patient is getting triangulated between family members—the one speaking to the physician and a family member being talked about. In Cole-Kelly et al's[20] study, the exemplar physicians were sensitive to the dangers of inappropriately colluding in a triangulated relationship with the patient and were very facile at avoiding those traps. The exemplars seemed to have an appreciation for the importance of understanding the concept of triangulation and to use it for their and the patient/family's advantage. The exemplars often explored family-oriented material during physical exams or while doing procedures, thus not using extra time for these areas of inquiry. Visits with a high family-oriented content occurred 19% of the time and family-oriented talk was low or absent in 52% of the visits. The visits that had the highest degree of family-oriented character were chronic illness visits and well-baby and child visits.

Asking some family-oriented questions can metaphorically bring the family into the exam room and provide a family context to the presenting problem.[21] Here are examples of family questions:

"Has anyone else in your family had this problem?" This question is often part of obtaining a genogram. It reveals not only whether there is a family history of the problem, but also how the family has responded to the problem in the past. The treatment used with one member of the family or in a previous generation may be a guide for the patient's approach to his/her illness or may describe how a patient does not want to proceed.

"What do your family members believe caused the problem or could treat the problem?" Family members often have explanatory models that strongly influence the patient's beliefs and behaviors regarding the health problem.[22] If the physician's treatment plan conflicts with what important family members believe or have recommended, it is unlikely the patient will comply.

"Who in your family is most concerned about the problem?" Sometimes another family member may be the one most concerned about the health problem and may be the actual person who really wants the patient to receive care. When the patient does seem concerned about the health problem or motivated to follow treatment recom-

mendations, finding out who is most concerned may be helpful in creating an effective treatment plan.

"Along with your illness (or symptoms), have there been any other recent changes in your family?" This question is a useful way to screen for other additional stressors, health problems, and changes in the patient's family and how it is affecting the patient.

"How can your family be helpful to you in dealing with this problem?" Discovering how family members can be a resource to the patient should be a key element of all treatment planning.

These questions can be integrated into a routine 15-minute office visit with an individual patient and provide valuable family information relevant to the problem.

Genograms

Genograms or family trees are one key to a family-oriented interview with an individual patient. They are the simplest and most efficient method for understanding the family context of a patient encounter[23] (Fig. 4.2) and provide a psychosocial "snapshot" of the patient. Genograms provides crucial information about genetic risks and any family history of serious illnesses. With advances in genetic research, a detailed genogram should be an essential component of every patient's medical evaluation and database. Ideally a genogram should integrate genetic and psychosocial information.

The genogram can be started at an initial visit and added to during subsequent encounters. It may be quite simple and only include the current household and family history of serious diseases or provide more detailed information about family events and relationships. When possible, the genogram should include family members' names, ages, marital status, significant illnesses, and dates of traumatic events, such as deaths. Computerized genogram programs are available so that the genogram can be integrated into an electronic medical record.

Obtaining a genogram can be a particularly effective way to understand the family context and obtain psychosocial information from a somatically focused or somatizing patient. These patients often present with multiple somatic complaints and try to keep the focus of the encounter on their physical symptoms and distress. They are challenging patients, and it is often difficult to obtain family or psychosocial information from them. Since obtaining a family history is considered a routine part of a medical evaluation, it can often provide access to more relevant psychosocial illness. It provides a way

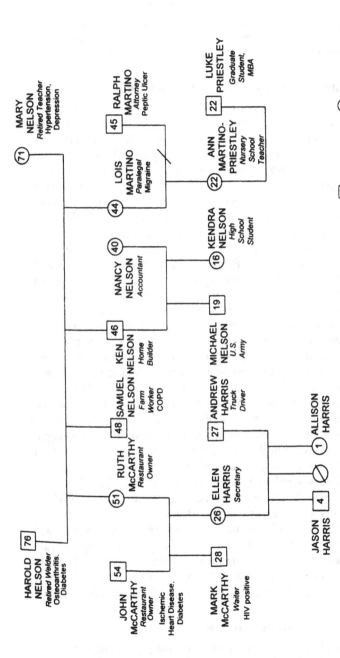

Fig. 2.2. Genogram.

Nelson family genogram: family members, occupations, chronic health problems. Symbols used: ▢, male, age 76; ◯, female, age 71; ⑦, female, age 71; ▢, marriage; ◯—▢, divorce; ⊘, deceased.

to step back from the presenting complaints to obtain a broader view of patients and their symptoms in a manner that is acceptable to the patients. The genogram can also be used to screen for substance abuse and family violence.[23]

Involving Family Members in Routine Office Visits

Routine visits, in which one or more family members are present, are common and may be initiated by the patient, family members, or the clinician. These visits allow clinicians to obtain the family members' perspective on the problem or the treatment plan and answer the family members' questions. Family members accompany the patient to office visits in approximately one third of all visits, and these visits last just a few minutes longer than other visits. In some situations, they may be more efficient and cost-effective than a visit with an individual patient because a family member can provide important information about the health problem, or the visit may answer questions that might later arise. Family members may serve various roles for the patients, including helping to communicate patient concerns to the doctor, helping patients to remember clinician recommendations, expressing concerns regarding the patient, and assisting patients in making decisions. Physicians report that the accompanying family members improve their understanding of the patient's problem and the patient's understanding of the diagnosis and treatment.

There are many situations when a family physician may want to invite another family member to the next office visit. Partners and spouses are routinely invited to prenatal visits. Fathers and co-parents should be invited to well-child visits, especially when the child has a health or behavior problem. Whenever there is a diagnosis of a serious medical illness or concern about adherence to medical treatments, it is helpful to invite the patient's spouse or other important family members to come for the next visit. Elderly couples are usually highly dependent on each other. It can be particularly effective and efficient to see them together for their routine visits. Each can provide information on how the other one is doing and help with implementation of treatment recommendations. Consulting with family members during a routine visit is advised whenever the health problem is likely to have a significant impact on other family members or when family members can be a resource in the treatment plan.

Principles of Family Interviewing

The principles of interviewing an individual patient also apply to interviewing families, but there are additional complexities. One must engage and talk with at least one additional person, and there is opportunity for interaction between the patient and family members. In general, the physician must be more active and establish clear leadership in a family interview. This may be as simple as being certain that each participant's voice is heard ("Mrs. Jones, we haven't heard from you about your concerns about your husband's illness. Can you share those?") or may entail acting as a traffic cop with a large and vocal family ("Jim, I know that you have some ideas about your mother's care, but I'd like to let your sister finish talking before we hear from you.").

When interviewing families, establishing rapport and an initial relationship with each family member is particularly important. In a family systems approach, this is known as joining. An essential component of joining is making some positive contact with each person present so that each feels valued and connected enough to the physician to participate in the interview. Family members have often been excluded from health care discussions and decisions, even when they are present. They may not expect to be included in the interview or to be asked to participate in decision making. By making contact and shaking hands with each person, the physician is making clear that everyone is encouraged to participate in the interview.

There are several other important reasons for joining with family members at the beginning of the interview. The physician often has an established relationship with the patient, but may not have one with other family members, who may feel either left out or that their role is merely that of an observer. One common example of this occurs commonly during hospital rounds when there is a family member by the bedside. The usual approach is to either ask family members to leave during the interview or to ignore them. This is disrespectful of families and fails to use family members as a resource. It is recommended that the physician greet and shake hands with each family member and find out something about each person. At a minimum, this may be the family member's relationship with the patient and involvement in the patient's health problems. It may also involve thanking them for their presence and help.

All the principles of good medical interviewing can be extended to family interviewing. It is helpful to encourage each family member to participate and to be as specific as possible when discussing problems. Individual and family strengths should be emphasized. Emotions that are present in any family member during the interview should be recognized and acknowledged: "Mr. Canapary, you look upset. Is there anything about your wife's health or her medical care that you are concerned about?" In addition, the physician must take an active role in blocking persistent interruptions and preventing one person from monopolizing the conversation.

Establishing a positive relationship with family members is particularly important and more challenging when there is conflict in the family. In these cases, a family member may assume that the physician has taken the side of the patient in the conflict. The physician must take extra steps to join with family members in conflict and establish one's neutrality. The goal in these situations is to develop an alliance with each family member and the patient without taking sides in the conflict. An exception to this goal is when family violence threatens and then safety must be the first priority.

In addition to establishing rapport and building a relationship through verbal communication, the physician can also make use of nonverbal strategies to enhance the relationship with the patient and family members. Just as it is important to be sure that the physician and an individual patient are in a comfortable sitting position and at eye level with one another, it is important also that other family members are sitting near enough that they can hear what's being said and be easily seen by the physician. This proximity will help the physician make eye contact with each person in the room.

Upon entering the room and seeing that one family member is sitting very far from the physician or isolated from other family members, the physician can gently motion the person to come closer to enhance the sense of everyone being included in the patient visit and being an important part of the encounter. Similarly, one family member might dominate both the verbal and nonverbal space in the encounter, making it difficult for the other family members to have as much involvement with the patient or physician. For these cases, the physician must "direct traffic," so all voices can be heard.

A physician who meets with multiple family members needs to learn how to avoid taking sides with one family member at the exclusion of another. It is very easy for the physician to unwittingly be pulled into unresolved conflicts between family members. In the case of an ill child, one parent may try to form a relationship with the physician that excludes the other parent. Or a wife can try to get the physician to side with her, hoping that the physician's alliance will bolster her position against her husband. To avoid getting caught in the middle of a triangle, the physician must listen to each member of the family but still remain neutral. Furthermore, the physician can assert that it won't be helpful to the family if the physician takes sides with one member against another. The physician can emphasize the importance of everyone working together as the most beneficial way to enhance the health care of the patient (Table 2.2).

Table 2.2. **Dos and Don'ts of Family Interviewing**

Dos
  Greet and shake hands with each family member.
  Affirm the importance of each person's contribution.
  Recognize and acknowledge any emotions expressed.
  Encourage family members to be specific.
  Maintain an empathic and noncritical stance with each person.
  Emphasize individual and family strengths.
  Block persistent interruptions.

Don'ts
  Don't let any one person monopolize the conversation.
  Don't allow family members to speak for each other.
  Don't offer advice or interpretations early in a family interview.
  Don't breach patient confidentiality.
  Don't take sides in a family conflict, unless some one's safety is
    involved.

Source: Adapted from McDaniel et al.[5]

Family Conferences

A family conference is usually a specially arranged meeting requested by the physician, patient, or family to discuss the patient's health problem or a family problem in more depth than can be addressed during a routine office visit (see Table 2.1). All the principles of family interviewing discussed previously are used in a family conference. However, a family conference is usually longer than most office visits and involves more planning and structure.

Every family physician should have the skills to convene and conduct a family conference or meeting. In a randomized controlled trial, Karofsky and colleagues[24] examined the impact of an initial family conference for new pediatric patients and their families through a randomized controlled trial. The families that received the family conference had fewer subsequent visits for health problems or to the emergency room and more visits for health supervision (well-child visits). This study suggests that family conferences may be cost-effective by reducing health care utilization.

Meeting with entire families is most important when diagnosing and treating life-threatening illnesses. Family members are usually eager to obtain information from the physician and want to know how they can be helpful. Most physicians meet with a patient's family at the time of a hospitalization to explain a diagnosis and treatment plan. A family meeting at the time of hospital discharge should be routine. Usually family members must assume the responsibility for the care of the patient and need detailed information about the patient's condition and follow-up treatment. One study of couples coping with a myocardial infarction found that the best predictor of the wife's emotional well-being 6 months after her husband's heart attack was whether she had an opportunity to meet and talk with his physician prior to discharge.[25] Under managed care, hospital stays have shortened dramatically, and patients are going home with significant health care needs that must be provided by family members or assisted by visiting nurses.

Family conferences should also be a routine part of palliative or end-of-life care, whether at home or in a hospice. Clarifying the patient's diagnosis and prognosis with the family can be very helpful for treatment planning. Family conferences are often essential to resolve conflicts about whether to move from curative to comfort care. Some family members may resist a patient's decision to stop chemotherapy or other medical treatments, often because they are not emotionally ready for the patient's death. If the decision can be discussed and emotional reactions shared in a family meeting, these problems or conflicts can be avoided. Finally, it is helpful to routinely meet with family members after a patient's death to answer questions, allow the sharing of grief, and assess how family members are coping. With large families or difficult problems, the physician may wish to ask a family therapist to help conduct the meeting.

Conducting a family conference requires skills in addition to those used when meeting with family members during a routine office visit. There are usually, but not always, more family members involved. A family assessment and some type of planned family intervention may be required. The reason for convening the family may involve difficult or conflictual issues, which require special skills to handle.

A detailed outline or blueprint for conducting a family conference has been described elsewhere.[5] Prior to meeting with the family, the physician should have a clear rational and initial plan for the conference. Here are the basic steps or phases of a family conference that can guide the physician.

Joining Phase

As discussed previously, it is particularly important to spend time to develop rapport with the family and get to know something about each family member at the beginning of the conference. This step is often neglected or given inadequate time by the inexperienced clinician. The family may want to discuss the problem or issue at the very outset, and the physician may lose the opportunity to join early and learn more about the family. The physician can stop the discussion of the problem and say, "I find it helpful to step back and learn a little bit more about each of you, before we discuss the problem." This joining phase, which may seem like social chat to the inexperienced, helps to create a sense of trust between the physician and family and an environment in which family members feel safe and supported. If the physician already knows the family well, this phase may be abbreviated but should not be eliminated.

Goal Setting

It is helpful to jointly establish goals for the conference with the family. This often begins with the physician's statement about why the family has been convened, for example, "to discuss your mother's illness and plans for further treatment." It is then useful to ask what the family wants to accomplish during the session. The family's goals may be quite different from the physician's, and they need to be respected and addressed. This is analogous to asking individual patients what they were hoping to achieve during a routine office visit.

Information Exchange

The physician may ask what the family knows about the patient's illness or problem. This is often more effective and informative than launching into a detailed description of the patient's problem without knowing the family's level of knowledge. It also allows the physician to directly address misunderstandings or misinformation and to identify whether family members have varying views of the problem. It is important to get the views of all the family members present, even if it's as simple as having a family member say he or she agrees with the others.

Obtaining further information about the family is usually very helpful in understanding the issues or problems that the family is dealing with. Gathering a more detailed genogram is an easy way to obtain this information, and families usually feel comfortable and often enjoy this process. It is crucial to identify family strengths and supports during the interview. These are the resources that the family members will use to cope with the problem or illness they are facing.

When conducting an interview with a large, conflictual, or enmeshed family, the physician usually needs to be more active than during interviews with individuals, directing the conversations between family members and managing arguments. Each family member should be encouraged to speak, and no one should be allowed to speak for someone else who is present. It is important not to let any one person monopolize the conversation, and to interrupt and solicit other family members' opinion on the topic.

Establishing a Plan

During this final phase, the physician should work with the family to develop a mutually agreed upon treatment plan and to clarify each person's role in carrying it out. The patient, physician, and family members should have input into the plan. For some families, this may require writing up a formal care plan that everyone can agree on.

Confidentiality

When working with family members, the family physician must maintain confidentiality with the patient. Prior to speaking with a family member, it is important that the physician is clear about what the patient feels can be shared and what, if anything, cannot be. A family member may bring up difficult or awkward concerns, but the physician may only disclose information the patient has approved (unless the patient is incompetent). In most cases, patients will agree that their care plan can be fully discussed with the family members. However, in family meetings involving adolescents or divorced parents, the rules for the meeting need to be clearly spelled out. The physician may remind families at the beginning: "John has agreed that I can talk with you about the options for his diabetes treatment. He, of course, will be the one who will make the final decisions, but we both think it will be helpful to have all of your thoughts about what may be best." Such discussions value both the doctor–patient relationship as well as the patient–family relationships. The positive support of these relationships is only one of the positive outcomes of well-crafted family meetings.

Conclusion

The aging of the population, advances in medical research, and changes in our health care delivery system will continue to have dramatic impact on family issues in health care. There are increasing demands on families to provide care for aged and chronically ill patients, often without adequate services and insurance reimbursements. Family caregiving has led to an increasing burden on family members and poor physical and mental health for many caregivers. The role of the family in end-of-life decision making is only beginning to be addressed. Health care proxy laws allow patients to identify an individual, usually a close family member, to make medical decisions if the patient is unable to, but little research has been done on how patients make these choices, what they discuss with their designated health care agent, and whether family members follow the wishes of the patient. Because of the genetic revolution, we will soon have the ability to screen or test for hundreds of genetic disorders, but the impact of this technology on families is just beginning to be examined. Genetic counseling needs to address not only the genetic risks of the individual but also the implications for other family members. More family research is need in each of these areas.

One of the unique and distinguishing characteristics of family medicine is its emphasis on the family. No other medical specialty has a family focus or uses a family-oriented approach. Under our changing health care system, there is increasing recognition of the importance and cost-effectiveness of involving the family in all aspects of medical care. New models of care are being developed that emphasize teamwork, prevention, and collaboration with patients and their families. A family-oriented approach will become increasingly valued and effective model in the 21st century.

References

1. Campbell TL. The family's impact on health: a critical review and annotated bibliography. Fam Syst Med 1986;4(2,3):135–328.
2. Doherty WA, Campbell TL. Families and health. Beverly Hills, CA: Sage, 1988.
3. House JS, Landis KR, Umberson D. Social relationships and health. Science 1988;241(4865):540–5.
4. Campbell TL, Patterson JM. The effectiveness of family interventions in the treatment of physical illness. J Marital Fam Ther 1995;21(4):545–83.
5. McDaniel SH, Campbell TL, Seaburn DB. Family-oriented primary care: a manual for medical providers 2nd Edition. New York: Springer-Verlag, 2003.
6. Doherty WJ, Baird MA. Family therapy and family medicine: toward the primary care of families. New York: Guilford, 1983.
7. Weihs K, Fisher L, Baird MA. Families, health and behavior. Institute of Medicine report. Washington, DC: National Academy Press, 2001.
8. Berkman LF, Leo-Summers L, Horwitz RI. Emotional support and survival after myocardial infarction. A prospective, population-based study of the elderly. Ann Intern Med 1992;117(12):1003–9.
9. Osterweis M, Solomon F, Green M. Bereavement: Reactions, consequences, and care. Washington DC: National Acadamy Press, 1984.
10. Kiecolt-Glaser JK, Fisher LD, Ogrocki P, Stout JC, Speicher CE, Glaser R. Marital quality, marital disruption, and immune function. Psychosom Med 1987;49(1):13–34.

11. Hooley JM, Orley J, Teasdale JD. Levels of expressed emotion and relapse in depressed patients. Br J Psychiatry 1986;148:642–7.
12. Kanter J, Lamb HR, Loeper C. Expressed emotion in families: a critical review [Review]. Hosp Community Psychiatry 1987;38(4):374–80.
13. Hooley JM, Richters JE. Expressed emotion: a developmental perspective. In: Cicchetti D, Toth SL, eds. Emotion, cognition, and representation. Rochester Symposium on Development Psychopathology. Rochester, NY: University of Rochester Press, 1995;133–66.
14. Fischmann-Havstad L, Marston AR. Weight loss maintenance as an aspect of family emotion and process. Br J Clin Psychol 1984;23(4):264–71.
15. Koenigsberg HW, Klausner E, Pelino D, Rosnick P. Expressed emotion and glucose control in insulin-dependent diabetes mellitus. Am J Psychiatry 1993;150(7):1114–5.
16. Ewart CK, Taylor CB, Kraemer HC, Agras WS. Reducing blood pressure reactivity during interpersonal conflict: effects of marital communication training. Behav Ther 1984;15(5):478–84.
17. Minuchin S, Baker L, Rosman BL, Liebman R, Milman L, Todd TC. A conceptual model of psychosomatic illness in children. Family organization and family therapy. Arch Gen Psychiatry 1975;32(8):1031–38.
18. McFarlane WR, Lukens E, Link B, Dushay R, Newmark M. Multi-family groups and psychoeducation in the treatment of schizophrenia. Arch Gen Psychiatry 1995;52(8):677–87.
19. Mittelman MS, Ferris SH, Shulman E, Steinberg G, Levin B. A family intervention to delay nursing home placement of patients with Alzheimer disease. A randomized controlled trial [see comments]. JAMA 1996;276(21):1725–31.
20. Cole-Kelly K, Yanoshik MK, Campbell J, Flynn SP. Integrating the family into routine patient care: a qualitative study. J Fam Pract 1998;47(6):440–5.
21. Cole-Kelly K, Seaburn D. Five areas of questioning to promote a family-oriented approach in primary care. Fam Syst Health 1999;17(3):348–54.
22. Wright LM, Bell JM, Rock BL. Smoking behavior and spouses: a case report. Fam Syst Med 1989;7(2):171–7.
23. McGoldrick M, Gerson R, Shellenberger S. Genograms: Assessment and intervention, 2nd ed. New York: W.W. Norton, 1999.
24. Karofsky PS, Rice RL, Hoornstra LL, Slater CJ, Kessinich CA, Goode JR. The effect of the initial family interview on a pediatric practice. Clin Pediatr 1991;30(5):290–4.
25. Fiske V, Coyne JC, Smith DA. Couples coping with myocardial infarction: an empirical reconsideration of the role of overprotectiveness. J Fam Psychol 1991;5(1):20–7.
26. McDaniel SH, Campbell TL, Hepworth J, Lorenz A. A manual of family-oriented primary care, 2nd edit. New York: Springer-Verlag. In Press.

3
Genetic Disorders

John W. Bachman

In family medicine, knowledge of genetics is useful in evaluating the risk a patient may have for a genetic disorder and to counsel patients about possible risks associated with any future childbearing. Today's family physician assumes many roles in managing genetic issues (Table 3.1). The explosion in science centering on genetics requires all primary care physicians to be aware of the pragmatic advances in this field.

The Basic Science of Genetics

There are 50,000 to 100,000 genes located in the 46 chromosomes of the human cell. Each gene is composed of one copy originating from the paternal side and the other from the maternal side. Genes are composed of DNA, and the ultimate products of most genes are proteins. The coding for a gene is its genotype. The physical result in the organism is its phenotype. It may not necessarily mean that the organism with the gene is expressed by its phenotype (recessive gene).

Most changes in the DNA of genes do not result in a disease; these are called polymorphisms. A change in the DNA of a gene that results in an abnormal protein that functions poorly or not at all is called a mutation. The same mutation in a gene does not necessarily produce the same physical findings in affected persons. This difference is called gene expression. Alleles are alternative forms of a gene at a specific location on a chromosome. A single allele for each locus

Table 3.1. **The Roles of Family Physicians in Genetic Medicine**

Identify individuals who are at increased risk for genetic disorders or who have a disorder

Use common prenatal genetic screening methods and effectively use genetic testing to care for individuals

Recognize the characteristics of common genetic disorders

Provide ongoing care for individuals with genetic disorders by monitoring health and coordinating referrals

Provide informed options about genetic issues to patients and their families

Be aware of genetic services for patients with various genetic disorders for appropriate referral

---

is inherited from each parent. Damage to DNA is corrected by DNA repair genes. Mutations of repair genes lead to an increased risk for cancer.

Types of Testing

Indirect Analysis–Linkage Analysis

This type of testing is used when the location of a gene is not known or it is too difficult to test for directly. It is used primarily in families and requires that one affected person be tested to determine whether the gene is located near some genetic material that can be measured, such as another gene or a segment of DNA. If a marker is found, it can be used in other family members to assess whether they might have the gene. (You find the gene by knowing the company it keeps.) A geneticist might order this testing in a patient if there is a clustering of a disease in the family.

Direct Mutation Analysis

This type of genetic analysis involves looking for the specific mutation on the gene by one of several techniques. Common ones include Southern blot analysis, multiplex polymerase chain reaction, and direct sequencing of the gene. It does not rely on testing other members of the family. A family physician or geneticist ordering this type of testing is looking for a specific mutation on a gene, usually because of observing a patient's phenotype. A limitation of this technique is that a disease may be caused by multiple mutations. An example is cystic fibrosis, which is the result of the loss of phenylalanine at position 508 in about 70% of cases. The other 30% of cases are caused by hundreds of other mutations on the gene. Therefore, it is unrealistic to check for all of them when screening an individual. Another issue is that sometimes more than two genes are involved and account for the same phenotype.

Molecular Cytogenetic Analysis

Chromosome rearrangements can be detected by fluorescence in situ hybridization (FISH). The technique involves preparing a fluorescent probe that identifies either the abnormal region (a visible color appears on examination) or a normal region (no color appears). The technique is quick but often requires follow-up studies.

Types of Genetic Disorders

The types of genetic disorders that the patients of family physicians may have can be classified as follows:

1. Chromosome disorders: These disorders are caused by the loss, gain, or abnormal arrangement of one or more chromosomes. Their frequency in the population is about 0.2%.
2. Mendelian disorders: These disorders are single-gene defects caused by a mutant allele at a single genetic locus. The transmission pattern is divided further into autosomal dominant, autosomal recessive, X-linked dominant, and X-linked recessive. Their frequency is about 0.35%.
3. Multifactorial disorders: These disorders involve interactions between genes and environmental factors. The nature of these interactions is poorly understood. It includes cancers, diabetes, and most other diseases that develop during a patient's life. The risks of transmission can be estimated empirically, and their estimated frequency in the population is about 5%.
4. Somatic genetic disorders: Mutations arise in somatic cells and are not inherited. They often give rise to malignancies. Although the mutation is not inherited, it often requires a genetic predisposition.
5. Mitochondrial disorders: These disorders arise from mutations in the genetic material in mitochondria. Mitochondrial DNA is transmitted through only the maternal line.

Each of these groups of disorders, except mitochondrial disorders, is discussed below.

Chromosome Abnormalities

Down Syndrome

The most frequent chromosome disorder (1 in 800 births in the United States) is the one associated with Down syndrome. Down syndrome is caused primarily by nondisjunction during development of the egg, with failure of a chromosome 21 pair to segregate during meiosis. The event is random. Another cause (3–4% of cases) is a robertsonian translocation, in which chromosome 21 attaches to another chromosome. Although the amount of genetic material is normal, the number of chromosomes is 45 instead of 46. The offspring of a parent with a robertsonian translocation have a 25% chance of having a Down syndrome karyotype. Karyotyping is required for all newborn children with Down syndrome to rule out robertsonian translocation. Another cause of Down syndrome (1–2% of cases) is nondisjunction after conception that leads to a mosaic pattern of inheritance, in which some cells are trisomy 21 and others are normal. A normal karyotype initially in a child with classic Down syndrome is possibly explained by mosaicism and requires chromosome analysis of other tissue. Down syndrome can be diagnosed during the prenatal period. The definitive tests are amniocentesis and chorionic villus sampling. Indications for either procedure are as follows[1]:

1. Robertsonian translocation and previous birth of a child with Down syndrome: For women younger than 30 years, the risk for recurrent Down syndrome is about 1%. For those older than 30, the risk is the same as that for other women of their age. The risk for recurrence in a patient with a robertsonian translocation is high.
2. Increasing maternal age: The risks for Down syndrome and other chromosome disorders according to maternal age are listed in Table 3.2. Prenatal diagnosis should be offered to women older than 35 years, who in fact comprise the largest group referred for genetic testing prenatally. About 25% of all Down syndrome births can be detected when age is used as a criterion.
3. Low serum levels of maternal α-fetoprotein: When testing for neural tube defects, another subset of pregnant women can be identified as being at risk for having a child with Down syndrome. Because the liver of a fetus with Down syndrome is immature, α-fetoprotein levels are lower than normal. Another 20% of fetuses with Down syndrome can be identified with this test (amniocentesis rate of 5% of a pregnant population being tested). The test also can be used to adjust patients older than age 35 years into a lower risk group.

Table 3.2. **Chromosome Abnormalities in Liveborn Infants, by Maternal Age[a]**

Maternal age (years)	Risk for Down syndrome	Total risk for chromosome abnormalities[b]
20	1/1667	1/526
21	1/1667	1/526
22	1/1429	1/500
23	1/1429	1/500
24	1/1250	1/476
25	1/1250	1/476
26	1/1176	1/476
27	1/1110	1/455
28	1/1053	1/435
29	1/1000	1/417
30	1/952	1/385
31	1/952	1/385
32	1/769	1/322
33	1/602	1/286
34	1/485	1/238
35	1/378	1/192
36	1/289	1/156
37	1/224	1/127
38	1/173	1/102
39	1/136	1/83
40	1/106	1/66
41	1/82	1/53
42	1/63	1/42
43	1/49	1/33
44	1/38	1/26
45	1/30	1/21
46	1/23	1/16
47	1/18	1/13
48	1/14	1/10
49	1/11	1/8

[a]Because sample size for some intervals is relatively small, 95% confidence limits are sometimes relatively large. Nonetheless, these figures are suitable for genetic counseling.

[b]47,XXX excluded for ages 20 to 32 years (data not available).

Source: Simpson,[16] by permission of Bailliere Tindall.

4. Triple test: The risk for Down syndrome can be ascertained by measuring the serum levels of α-fetoprotein, estrogen, and human chorionic gonadotropin (hCG). The serum hCG level is higher and that of unconjugated estriols is lower in a pregnant woman whose

fetus has Down syndrome. Detection rates of 60%, with an amniocentesis rate of 5% of a pregnant population being tested, have been reported.

All biochemical tests used for screening can produce false-positive results. It is important to confirm gestational age with ultrasonography before proceeding with amniocentesis to evaluate abnormal serum findings. Generally, routine screening exclusively with multiple biochemical markers is not recommended. None of the screening studies can guarantee that a child does *not* have Down syndrome. The definitive diagnostic study is amniocentesis or chorionic villus sampling. The advantage of chorionic villus sampling is earlier detection of Down syndrome so an abortion can be performed earlier during the pregnancy. The disadvantage is that the sampling is not useful for detecting neural tube defects.

When counseling patients, a family physician should discuss the cost of the studies, the risks, and the concerns of the parents. During a discussion about children with Down syndrome, important points that should be made include the 33% chance of cardiac abnormalities, the presence of other congenital conditions, intellectual development to the level of the third to ninth grade, and the ability of most children to leave home and live independently as adults. Although it once was thought that only women who would have an abortion should undergo testing for Down syndrome, it is acceptable to use the tests to identify a high-risk pregnancy that may require care at a tertiary medical center.

At birth, a child with Down syndrome is identified on the basis of the following physical examination findings: hypotonia, craniofacial features of brachycephaly, oblique palpebral fissures, epicanthal folds, broad nasal bridge, protruding tongue, and low-set ears. The child may have Brushfield spots; short, broad fingers; a single flexion crease in the hand (the so-called simian crease, which is present in 30% of children with Down syndrome and about 5% of normal children); and a wide space between the first two toes. About a third of the children have recognizable congenital heart disease, and the risk of duodenal atresia and tracheoesophageal fistula is increased. It is important to recognize congenital heart disease during the newborn period, and echocardiography is mandatory. Irreversible pulmonary hypertension with no recognizable signs can develop by 2 months. Ophthalmologic examination for cataracts, hearing tests, thyroid tests, and a complete blood cell count for leukemoid reaction should be performed.

An effective method has been described for informing parents that their child has Down syndrome. The basic principle is to tell both parents as soon as possible, with the baby present, in a quiet, private room. The child is referred to by name, and the information is provided by a credible person who can provide a balanced point of view. This person then gives the parents his or her telephone number should they have additional questions, and the family is given time to absorb the information. Other suggestions include providing information about the National Down Syndrome Society (1-800-221-4602) and having other parents of children with Down syndrome visit the new parents.

During the first 5 years of life, it is important to check for hypothyroidism annually, evaluate vision and hearing at 6-month to 1-year intervals, and provide special education. Growth charts are available online.[2] All children with Down syndrome should stay with the family, and most can be mainstreamed into kindergarten. It is important to use standard measures for Down syndrome to monitor growth and development. A child with Down syndrome often has a problem with verbal learning in school and does much better with visual learning. Resources for enhancing education are available from the National Association for Down Syndrome. A comprehensive resource for health supervision is available.[3] Before children with Down syndrome participate in sports, instability of the atlantodens must be assessed on cervical radiographs. Children who require intubation also may need evaluation. How frequent these radiographs should be obtained is debatable. No child has become paralyzed in the Special Olympics, and 90% of children in whom paralysis developed because of instability showed symptoms during the preceding month.

Most people with Down syndrome are able to leave home, work, and form relationships. Counseling them about contraceptive measures is appropriate. Alzheimer disease occurs in 25% of adults with Down syndrome.

Turner Syndrome

Turner syndrome has an incidence of about 1 in 2000 births.[4] The syndrome involves errors in one of the X chromosomes, such as the absence of one X chromosome (60% of cases), a structural abnormality of an X chromosome (20% of cases), or mosaicism involving the X chromosome of at least one cell line (20% of cases). Cases now are often discovered with prenatal amniocentesis and ultrasonography.

Heart Lesions

Many Turner syndrome patients have left-sided heart lesions, such as postductal coarctation (up to 20%) and bicuspid aortic valves (up to 50%), with or without stenosis. With time, distention of the ascending aorta may develop, leading to damage, possible dilation, dissection, and premature atherosclerosis. Echocardiography is recommended during infancy and the second decade of life. Bicuspid valves are an indication for prophylactic treatment for subacute bacterial endocarditis.

Bone Abnormalities

Osteoporosis is common with Turner syndrome, and calcium supplementation is important. Medical therapy may be indicated depending on bone density. Other skeletal characteristics include micrognathia, short metacarpals, genu valgum, scoliosis, and a square, stocky appearance.

Puberty

Oocytes degenerate by the time of birth in most cases of Turner syndrome. Between the ages of 12 and 15, puberty is induced with estrogens, and after 12 months progesterone is added to the regimen. Pregnancy has occurred in spontaneously menstruating patients. These patients usually have a mosaic pattern. In medical centers that specialize in in vitro fertilization, pregnancy rates of 50% to 60% have been reported with the use of both sister and anonymous donors.

Stature

Failure of growth occurs in virtually all patients with Turner syndrome. Often intrauterine growth failure is mild, height increases normally until age 3, growth velocity is progressive until age 14, and the adolescent growth phase is long. The short stature responds to treatment with growth hormone. It should begin when the stature is less than the fifth percentile (usually at age 2–5 years). Estrogen treatment may commence in adolescence.

Other Common Problems

Glucose intolerance, hearing loss over time, hypothyroidism (up to 50% by the time of adulthood), and congenital urinary tract abnormalities are more common among patients with Turner syndrome (35–70%) than in the general population. Fetal lymphedema may cause webbing of the neck, a low posterior hairline, and auricular malrotation.

Studies to consider for patients with Turner syndrome include chromosome karyotyping, thyroid function tests (annually), a baseline evaluation of the kidneys, and echocardiography.

Klinefelter Syndrome

Klinefelter syndrome is characterized by a 47,XXY karyotype.[3,4] It has an incidence of 1.7 in 1000 male infants. The disorder usually is diagnosed at puberty or during an infertility evaluation. In adolescents, its characteristics include gynecomastia (40%), small testicles (<2.5 cm long), tall stature, and an arm span that is greater than the person's height. Klinefelter syndrome is the most common cause of hypogonadism in males; testosterone levels are about half the normal value. The follicle-stimulating hormone and lactate dehydrogenase levels are increased. Treatment includes testosterone and occasionally mastectomy for gynecomastia.

Other Chromosome Abnormalities

Trisomy 18 is the second most common trisomy (1 in 8000 births).[3,4] Fewer than 10% of affected infants survive to age 1 year. Trisomy 13, the third most common trisomy, has an incidence of 1 in 20,000 births. Fifty percent of affected children die during the first month, and fewer than 5% survive beyond age 3. Cri du chat syndrome is due to a deletion involving chromosome 5. The incidence is 1 in 20,000 births. The clinical features include severe mental retardation, hypotonia, and a kitten-like cry. Life expectancy is the same as that for other patients with similar IQs.

Mendelian Disorders

Genogram

Knowledge of the family history is a powerful weapon for preventing premature death.[5] The first step in detecting a mendelian disorder involves constructing a genogram of the family history. Although genograms are used by fewer than 20% of family physicians, they are useful for showing patterns of genetic inheritance. One study indicated that three fourths of patients referred for genetic counseling had another significant family disorder that could affect pregnancy. Reports have demonstrated that 90% of doctors are able to interpret data from a genogram written by other colleagues. To save time, a medical assistant can initially question a patient about the family history of genetic disorders before a physician obtains a complete medical history. The information collected includes the following:

1. Demographic data: the names of relatives and their birth dates, ages, sexes, spontaneous abortions, places of residence, and dates of death.
2. Medical disorders: a listing of the diseases experienced by family members
3. Social factors: relationships and the nature of these relationships
4. Other data: previous family crises

When a genogram is constructed, squares are used to represent male members and circles to represent female members. Three generations should be represented, and each generation is on a horizontal row. A first-degree relative is a parent, sibling, or child. A second-degree relative is an aunt, uncle, nephew, niece, grandparent, or grandchild.

Dominant Disorders

With classic dominant inheritance, the affected person has a parent with the disorder. The parent usually mates with someone who does not have the genetic disorder, and the offspring have a 50% chance of having the disorder. Typically, predisposition for the disorder is carried on one chromosome, and expression of the disorder is modified by the chromosome makeup of the other parent. The dominant condition usually does not alter the ability to reproduce but tends to alter materials that provide structure to a body. Examples of dominant disorders include Marfan syndrome, Huntington disease, neurofibromatosis, achondroplasia, and familial hypercholesterolemia. About 6% of cases of breast cancer are inherited dominantly. For construction of a genogram, an excellent screening question for dominant disorders is, "Has anyone in your family had a serious disorder during adolescence or middle age?" Diseases that seem to be present in each generation tend to be dominant.

Recessive Disorders

With classic recessive-disorder inheritance, both mates have a gene for the disorder. The offspring have a 25% chance of having a normal gene pattern, a 50% chance of being a carrier, and a 25% chance of having the disorder. Carriers tend to have a reproductive advantage in certain environments; for example, sickle cell trait carriers are more resistant to falciparum malaria than noncarriers. The disorders tend to involve enzymes, and siblings who have the disorder tend to have the same severity because there is no modifying gene as in a dominant disorder. If untreated, recessive disorders tend to cause death at an early age.

Screening questions that are useful for revealing recessive disorders include "Has anyone in your family had stillbirths?" and "Has anyone in your family had children who died or were seriously ill during early childhood?" An important consideration when screening for recessive disorders[6] is to inquire about the nationality of the patient. Certain nationalities are associated with recessive disorders. For example, in patients of Caribbean, Latin American, Mediterranean, or African descent, hemoglobin testing should be performed to screen for sickle cell anemia or thalassemia disorders. Patients of Ashkenazi Jewish origin should be screened for Tay-Sachs disease and possibly Gaucher disease (1 in 450 births). There are exceptions to this tendency. For example, hemochromatosis is a very common recessive disorder and is often frequently missed because the symptoms occur late in life.

In addition to the medical history, laboratory screening tests performed in the newborn detect recessive disorders. States require that many of these tests be performed. Examples are phenylketonuria, galactosemia, congenital adrenal hyperplasia, and hemoglobinopathy tests. The ideal time for conducting these laboratory studies is 72 hours after birth, although with early hospital dismissal of newborns, this timing is difficult. The American Academy of Pediatrics recommends that screening tests be performed in all infants before dismissal from the hospital. If the infant is dismissed less than 24 hours after birth, the screening tests should be repeated before the infant is 2 weeks old. Many medical clinics recommend rescreening if dismissal occurs at 48 hours. The diagnoses of phenylketonuria and hypothyroidism may be missed if the infant is not retested after early dismissal. In some states, other newborn screening tests are performed to detect galactosemia (incidence of 1 in 50,000 births; it involves a defect in the enzyme for converting glucose to galactose), hemoglobinopathies, and congenital adrenal hyperplasia. Follow-up data for children with abnormal screening results have been published.[7]

Newborns who become progressively more ill usually are thought to have a septic condition. An inborn error of metabolism should be considered in a newborn who vomits and becomes progressively comatose. Also, it is important to remember that a mother who has phenylketonuria should be placed on a rigorous phenylalanine-free diet when pregnant to ensure that her condition does not cause mental retardation in the fetus. Ideally, this diet is started during the pre-conception period.

Cystic Fibrosis

A recessive disorder currently discussed widely is cystic fibrosis.[8,9] Nearly 30,000 people in the United States have this disorder. It is carried by about 1 in 25 Caucasians in the U.S., and these carriers often do not have a family history of cystic fibrosis. The clinical characteristics of cystic fibrosis include pancreatic insufficiency (85% of patients), pulmonary disease characterized by recurrent infections and bronchiectasis, and failure to grow. In more than 60% of patients, the diagnosis is made during the first year of life. Interestingly, the diagnosis is made in 5% of patients after age 15 years. Most authorities believe that early diagnosis prevents pulmonary damage in early life, but, currently, routine screening of infants is not recommended.[10] The diagnosis is based on the concentration of chloride in sweat being greater than 60 mEq/L and clinical suspicion of the disease. Improvements in antibiotics, physiotherapy, and nutrition have increased the average age of survival from 4 years in 1960 to 30 years in 1995. Current advances in treatment include agents that break down mucus and trials for gene therapy. The mucus produced in a patient with cystic fibrosis provides an excellent medium for *Pseudomonas* and other bacteria that damage lungs. Cross-infection has led to cystic fibrosis organizations' discouraging camps for patients and developing guidelines for limiting this problem. The gene associated with cystic fibrosis was identified in 1989 on chromosome 7 and encodes the protein cystic fibrosis transmembrane conductance regulator, which is a chloride channel in cells. The failure of this channel to work properly causes excess chloride in sweat and changes in fluid balance, which in turn cause thickened mucus in the lungs. The most common defect in cystic fibrosis cells is the absence of phenylalanine in the protein (deletion). Testing is recommended for patients with a family history of cystic fibrosis and their partners. There are more than 150 mutations of the cystic fibrosis gene, and testing can detect 85% of the carriers.

Multifactorial Disorders

Neural Tube Defects

Neural tube defects (NTDs) are the disorders most commonly screened for prenatally.

Physiology

α-Fetoprotein is synthesized in the yolk sac, gastrointestinal tract, and liver. The protein enters the amniotic fluid through urination, secretions, and transudation from blood vessels, and small amounts leak into the maternal serum.

Incidence

The incidence of NTDs is 1 to 2 in 1000 births. A family history of NTDs and diabetes in the mother increase the risk significantly. If the mother's diet is supplemented with folic acid before conception, the incidence of NTDs decreases. These defects are associated with high mortality, high morbidity, and long-term developmental disability.

Screening

Of every 1000 pregnant females who are tested at 16 to 18 weeks' gestation in the U.S., about 25 to 50 have increased levels of maternal serum α-fetoprotein (msAFP) and 40 to 50 have low levels.[9,10] The mothers with high levels of msAFP can undergo ultrasonography to determine gestational age or the presence of a multiple gestation or significant abnormality. An alternative is to repeat the test within 1 to 2 weeks for mothers with abnormally high or low levels of the protein. If the repeat studies confirm the previous abnormal results, ultrasonography is performed. After screening with ultrasonography, about 17 of the patients with increased levels of msAFP and 20 to 30 of those with low levels have no findings that explain the abnormal values. Amniocentesis should be performed in these patients. Of the 17 patients with high levels, one or two have a fetus with a significant NTD, whereas 1 in 65 of those with a low msAFP have a fetus with a chromosome abnormality (1 in 90 chance of Down syndrome). For a pregnant female with an abnormally high msAFP level and a fetus with no NTD, the risk of stillbirth, low birth weight, neonatal death, and congenital anomalies is increased. Excellent summaries are available.[11]

Other Disorders

The overall risk for recurrent cleft lip, with or without cleft palate, is 4% if a sibling or parent has the abnormality and 10% if it is present in two previous siblings. Lip pits or depressions on the lower lip of a newborn may be the manifestation of an autosomal-dominant trait; the recurrence rate for a sibling is 50%.

Generally, the incidence of multifactorial disorders is less than 5%. The incidence of recurrence is 2% to 5% for cardiac anomalies, 1% to 2% for tracheoesophageal fistula, 1% to 2% for diaphragmatic hernia, 6% to 10% for hypospadias, and 4% to 8% for hip dislocation.

General Considerations in Counseling Patients

In North America about 8% of pregnancies meet the criteria for performing amniocentesis or chorionic villus sampling. The following are basic points for prenatal testing:

1. All patients have the right to receive information about the genetic risk associated with a pregnancy. It allows parents to make an informed choice about having a child with an abnormality.
2. All patients have the right to refuse testing. What a patient decides to do about any given risk factor is entirely up to the patient. Genetic testing is voluntary, except for what a state requires (e.g., neonatal screening for phenylketonuria, hypothyroidism, and other inborn errors of metabolism).
3. Referral to a geneticist is useful for difficult cases or patients with complex or unusual genetic disorders.
4. Genetic screening is not expected to detect all genetic disorders in a given population.

Cancer and Genetics

Certain families have an increased risk for specific cancers.[12] Many of these families have an identifiable gene associated with the disorder. Possession of the gene does not automatically mean that cancer will develop in the patient. Most genes can be altered by environmental factors and by other genes. In some families a defective gene is inherited, such as for retinoblastoma. With time there is a somatic mutation of the other normal copy of the gene. With colorectal carcinoma there is a multistep process in which a cell mutates and forms a family of abnormal cells, one of which mutates to form another cell line. Over time, these accumulated multiple mutations form a cell line that is cancer. Consequently, a risk can be predicted on the basis of the history of the gene being found in other families. One of the most important concepts to remember is that if an abnormal cancer gene is found in a patient who is not a member of a family with a history of cancer, there is minimal evidence for determining risk for the patient for that cancer. Most single-gene disorders that predispose to cancer are rare. Colon cancer and breast cancer, described below, are exceptions to this rule.

Colon Cancer

Inherited colon cancer represents 5% to 10% of colon cancer cases and about 30% of adult genetic referrals. It is reassuring to family members that no matter how extensive the family history of colon cancer, the risk for development of colon cancer never exceeds 50% in a family member.

Familial Adenomatous Polyposis (Gardner Syndrome)

Familial adenomatous polyposis has an incidence of 1 in 10,000 and makes up less than 1% of colon cancers. It is caused by having an autosomal-dominant gene located on chromosome 5 (*APC* gene). Predictive testing of first-degree relatives is appropriate, and those who have the gene need colon studies starting at age 12 years. Once several polyps are found, colon resection is recommended. Regular surveillance afterward is needed to assess potential cancers in the upper intestinal tract.

Hereditary Nonpolyposis Colon Cancer

Most observers believe that hereditary nonpolyposis colon cancer accounts for 2% of colon cancers and is the result of a defect on *hMSH2* found on chromosome 2 or four other genes. They are autosomal dominant. All genes in this group are mismatch repair genes. The genes function in repairing abnormal DNA. Consequently, for a tumor to appear it must be altered and the genes for repair absent. This is called the "two-hit hypothesis." Colonoscopy is the preferred method of screening at intervals of 18 months to 3 years depending on the family history. Suggested surveillance guidelines can be found in the literature.[13]

Breast Cancer

Among all women with breast cancer, 20% to 30% have at least one relative with breast cancer. Among these cases, 5% to 10% are caused by mutations in *BRCA1* and *BRCA2* genes. Inherited breast cancer has the clinical features of younger age at onset (less than 45), bilaterality, and cancer at other sites. The genes are tumor-suppressor genes (they repair damaged DNA), and the loss of both alleles is required for the initiation of tumors. Testing is reasonable in patients with the following:

1. One first-degree relative age 30 years or less with breast cancer or a male relative with breast cancer.
2. Two first-degree relatives with breast cancer, one of whom is younger than 50 years or both are younger than 60 years, or one has bilateral breast cancer or both have ovarian cancer.
3. One first-degree relative with breast cancer and one first-degree relative with ovarian cancer.
4. One first-degree relative and one second-degree relative with breast cancer if the sum of their ages at onset is less than 110 or one has bilateral disease.
5. Two second-degree relatives with breast cancer if the sum of their ages is 60 or less.
6. *BRCA1* gene: The first identified gene for breast cancer is located on chromosome 17, and more than 600 mutations have been detected. A woman carrying a mutation is estimated to have a 56% to 87% lifetime risk of having breast cancer and a 15% to 45% chance of having a lifetime risk of ovarian cancer.
7. *BRCA2* gene: The second gene for breast cancer was detected in 1995 and has more than 150 mutations. The lifetime risks for development of breast cancer (37–87%) and ovarian cancer (10–20%) are somewhat less than the risks associated with the *BRCA1* gene.

Human Genome

On June 26, 2000, the Human Genome Project and Celera Genomics jointly announced that the human genome had been sequenced. The development of genetic information brought on by the sequencing of the human genome is accelerating. How useful is knowledge about sequencing of the human genome to clinicians? It certainly bodes well for a single mendelian gene. However, most common diseases rely on several genes. The situation has been described well by Holtzman and Marteau[14]:

It would be revolutionary if we could determine the genotypes of the majority of people who will get common diseases. The complexity of the genetics of common diseases casts doubt on whether accurate prediction will ever be possible. Alleles at many different gene loci will increase the risk of certain diseases only when they are inherited with alleles at other loci, and only in the presence of specific environmental or behavioral factors. Moreover, many combinations of predisposing alleles, environmental factors, and behavior could all lead to the same pathogenic effect.

The basic science of the human genome is not yet being applied in the family physician's office, but its use will follow predictable patterns. The first stage is identification of a gene that causes an illness. The second stage is development of methods to do genetic testing in a physician's practice. With the ability to identify the gene come the issues of carrier testing, presymptomatic genetic screening, and odds of the gene being fully expressed. Currently, gene therapy for altered DNA is restricted to protocols.

Current research efforts revolve around single nucleotide polymorphisms (SNPs, or "snips"). These are fragments of DNA that vary by a single DNA alteration. There are thousands of these fragments, and they make up less than 0.1% of a human's DNA. They determine the essential differences between individuals. The first application of SNPs is in drug use. For example, Glaxo developed a medication called alosetron hydrochloride (Lotronex) for irritable bowel syndrome. It was withdrawn from the market because 43 people had side effects. By analyzing DNA from patients who had side effects, it is hoped that the DNA difference that led to the side effect could be determined. Testing patients for this difference before the drug is used might lead to safe use. The use of SNPs to determine which patients are susceptible to medication reactions will probably be the first application that family physicians will use widely. Testing most likely will be done with a biochip made up of DNA strands; when a patient's DNA is compared with the chip, differences will be highlighted, pointing to significant problems with prescribing medication or eventually subtyping diseases such as diabetes and autoimmune diseases.

Finally, it is important to consider that genetic sequencing of pathogens will yield promising treatments. *Mycobacterium tuberculosis* and *Treponema pallidum* are examples of organisms whose genomes are now known.

Web Sites of Value

A reasonable way of keeping up with innovations is to use the Internet. The following sites are useful:

The Human Genome Projects Information: *http://www.ornl.gov/hgmis.*

A useful site that includes maps, genes, and diseases is the GENAT-LAS query: *http://bisance.citi2.fr/GENATLAS/menu_an.html*

PubMed has extensive resources for genetics[15]: *http://www.ncbi.nlm. nih.gov/Genbank/index.html*. At this time the site is more useful to basic science. It has *Molecular Biology of the Cell,* a textbook, online.

Montana State publishes a series of education topics quarterly. It is located at *http://www.mostgene.org/gd/gdlist.htm*.

George Washington University produces lectures of high quality in its Frontiers in Clinical Genetics: *http://www.frontiersingenetics. com/main.htm*.

OMIM—Online Mendelian Inheritance in Man: *http://www.ncbi.nlm. nih.gov/Omim*. The site tends to be comprehensive but focuses on basic sciences.

A society-based site for education, National Coalition of Health Professional Education in Genetics: *http://www.nchpeg.org*.

GeneClinics: *http://www.geneclinics.org*. An excellent all-around site for information that is current and well supported for clinicians.

GeneTests: *http://www.genetests.org/*. This site has materials and directories for genetic testing.

The genetics and rare conditions site of the University of Kansas has information for patients, *http://www.kumc.edu/gec/geneinfo.html*, and providers, *http://www.kumc.edu/gec/prof/geneelsi.html*.

Acknowledgment

Portions of this chapter were previously published in Bachman JW. Medical genetics. In: Breslow L, ed. Encyclopedia of public health. New York: Macmillan Publishers 2001, with permission of the publisher.

References

1. Layman LC. Essential genetics for the obstetrician/gynecologist. Obstet Gynecol Clin North Am 2000;27:555–66.
2. Richards G. Growth charts for children with Down syndrome. Available at *www.growthcharts.com/index.htm*.
3. Cunniff C, Frias JL, Kaye C, et al. Health supervision for children with Down syndrome. Pediatrics 2001;107:442–9.
4. Saenger P. Turner's syndrome. N Engl J Med 1996;335:1749–54.
5. Jolly W, Froom J, Rosen MG. The genogram. J Fam Pract 1980;10: 251–5.

6. Buist NR, Tuerck JM. The practitioner's role in newborn screening. Pediatr Clin North Am 1992;39:199–211.
7. Pass KA, Lane PA, Fernhoff PM, et al. US newborn screening system guidelines II: follow-up of children, diagnosis, management, and evaluation. Statement of the Council of Regional Networks for Genetic Services (CORN). J Pediatr 2000;137(suppl):S1–46.
8. Robinson P. Cystic fibrosis. Thorax 2001;56:237–41.
9. Welsh MJ, Smith AE. Cystic fibrosis. Sci Am 1995;273:52–9.
10. Genetic testing for cystic fibrosis. NIH Consensus Statement 1997;15: 1–37.
11. Congenital disorders. Screening for neural tube defects—including folic acid/folate prophylaxis. In: Guide to clinical preventive services, 2nd ed. 2001. Available at *www.cpmcnet.columbia.edu/texts/gcps/gcps0052.html*.
12. Weitzel JN. Genetic counseling for familial cancer risk. Hosp Pract 1996;31:57–69.
13. Cole TR, Sleightholme HV. ABC of colorectal cancer. The role of clinical genetics in management. Br Med J 2000;321:943–6.
14. Holtzman NA, Marteau TM. Will genetics revolutionize medicine? N Engl J Med 2000;343:141–4.
15. McEntyre J, Lipman D. PubMed: bridging the information gap. Can Med Assoc J 2001;164:1317–9.
16. Simpson JL. Screening for fetal and genetic abnormalities. Baillieres Clin Obstet Gynaecol 1991;5:675–96.

4
Care of the Obese Patient

Michael T. Railey

An estimated 97 million adults in the United States are overweight or obese. Obesity is the most common nutritional disease of the Western world.[1] The number of overweight Americans has increased from 20% to 34% over the last 10 to 12 years, with one half of adults overweight and one of three obese.[2] Twenty-five percent of children and adolescents are also considered obese.[2,3] In the United States, the prevalence of obesity is highest among African-American women (48.6%) and Mexican-American women (46.7%).[2] The reasons for this are multifactorial and strongly imply that effective treatments will have to include management plans that encompass cultural awareness. Management of obesity is individualized, complicated, and often frustrating for both patient and physician.[4] Obesity is associated with numerous health risks. Excess body weight increases the risk of developing cardiovascular disease, hypertension, diabetes, and many other diseases[5-8] (Table 4.1). The direct health care costs of treating obesity and its related diseases have been estimated to be $45.8 billion per year.[1,9,10] Indirect costs due to loss of income amounts to another $23 billion annually.[9]

Etiology

Obesity is a very complex and heterogeneous disease; its pathogenesis involves genetic influences combined with an imbalance between caloric intake and energy output. Other elements that play an addi-

Table 4.1. **Health Complications of Obesity**

Hypertension
Diabetes
Cancer (breast, possibly colon, others)
Dyslipidemias
Arthritis
Depression
Cholelithiasis
Coronary Artery Disease
Obstructive sleep apnea

tional role in the development of obesity include race, age, gender, and environmental and psychosocial factors. More specific evidence is rapidly accumulating, in the study of the genetic components of obesity. Researchers have identified an appetite suppressor released from fat cells called leptin.[11] Further interest has focused on the *Ob* or "obesity" gene and its subtypes.[11] The current model for a clinical approach to this difficult-to-treat condition is that of a chronic disease with a definite genetic influence requiring treatment on multiple levels, predominantly directed at environmental and behavioral changes.

Diagnosis

The measurement of height and weight should be a part of every comprehensive patient visit. Initially, the Hamwi principle can be used to estimate ideal body weight (IBW) in screening for endogenous obesity.[9] IBW is estimated using this principle (Table 4.2). When IBW is exceeded, body mass index (BMI) should also be calculated or determined using Figure 4.1; this value is recorded in the permanent medical record for future reference.[5] The calculation can be made by dividing the patient's weight in kilograms by the square of the height in inches as a BMI greater than or equal to 30. Morbid obesity is considered a BMI of 40 or more.[12]

Table 4.2. **Determination of Ideal Body Weight**

Men: 106 lbs for 5 feet in height plus 6 lbs for each additional inch
Women: 100 lbs for 5 feet in height plus 5 lbs for each additional inch
Light frame: reduce estimate by 10%
Heavy frame: add 10%

Height (Feet and Inches)

Weight(Pounds)	5'0"	5'1"	5'2"	5'3"	5'4"	5'5"	5'6"	5'7"	5'8"	5'9"	5'10"	5'12"	6'0"	6'1"	6'2"	6'3"	6'4"
100	20	19	18	18	17	17	16	16	15	15	14	14	14	13	13	12	12
105	21	20	19	19	18	17	17	16	16	15	15	15	14	14	13	13	13
110	21	21	20	19	19	18	18	17	17	16	16	15	15	15	14	14	13
115	22	22	21	20	20	19	19	18	17	17	17	16	16	15	15	14	14
120	23	23	22	21	21	20	19	19	18	18	17	17	16	16	15	15	15
125	24	24	23	22	22	21	20	20	19	18	18	17	17	16	16	16	15
130	25	25	24	23	22	22	21	21	20	19	19	18	18	17	17	16	16
135	26	26	25	24	23	22	22	21	21	20	19	19	18	18	17	17	16
140	27	26	26	25	24	23	23	22	21	21	20	20	19	18	18	17	17
145	28	27	27	26	25	24	23	23	22	21	21	20	20	19	19	18	18
150	29	28	27	27	26	25	24	23	23	22	22	21	20	20	19	19	18
155	30	29	28	27	27	26	25	24	24	23	22	22	21	20	20	19	19
160	31	30	29	28	27	27	26	25	24	24	23	22	22	21	21	20	19
165	32	31	30	29	28	27	27	26	25	24	24	23	22	22	21	21	20
170	33	32	31	30	29	28	27	27	26	25	24	24	23	22	22	21	21
175	34	33	32	31	30	29	28	27	27	26	25	24	24	23	22	22	21
180	35	34	33	32	31	30	29	28	27	27	26	25	24	24	23	22	22
185	36	35	34	33	32	31	30	29	28	27	27	26	25	24	24	23	23
190	37	36	35	34	33	32	31	30	29	28	27	26	26	25	24	24	23
195	38	37	36	35	33	32	31	31	30	29	28	27	26	26	25	24	24
200	39	38	37	35	34	33	32	31	30	30	29	28	27	26	26	25	24
205	40	39	37	36	35	34	33	32	31	30	29	29	28	27	26	26	25
210	41	40	38	37	36	35	34	33	32	31	30	29	28	28	27	26	26
215	42	41	39	38	37	36	35	34	33	32	31	30	29	28	28	27	26
220	43	42	40	39	38	37	36	35	34	33	32	31	30	29	28	27	27
225	44	43	41	40	39	37	36	35	34	33	32	31	31	30	29	28	27
230	45	43	42	41	39	38	37	36	35	34	33	32	31	30	30	29	28
235	46	44	43	42	40	39	38	37	36	35	34	33	32	31	30	29	29
240	47	45	44	43	41	40	39	38	36	35	34	33	32	31	31	30	29
245	48	46	45	43	42	41	40	38	37	36	35	34	33	32	31	31	30
250	49	47	46	44	43	42	40	39	38	37	36	35	34	33	32	31	30

Fig. 4.1. Determination of body mass index.

Deposits of fat in the upper body leading to particular configurations also put an individual at higher risk for metabolic abnormalities and the ravages of the obesity syndrome.[5] Sometimes referred to as "apple or pear" configurations, the waist to hip ratio (WHR) has been the most widely accepted practical method of classifying body fat distribution.[13] Measuring the smallest circumference below the rib cage and above the navel as the waist circumference, and the widest circumference at the posterior of the buttocks over the greater trocanters as the hip circumference, a ratio (waist to hip) is obtained. A WHR of 0.95 or less for men and 0.85 or less in women are the normal cutoff points.[1,5,13] Elevated measurements indicate increased risk for associated illnesses (see Table 4.1).[5,9,13]

There are rare secondary causes of obesity, which must be considered prior to constructing a treatment plan. These secondary causes include hypothalamic obesity due to trauma, malignancy, inflammatory disease, Cushing syndrome, growth hormone deficiency, hypogonadism, hypothyroidism, polycystic ovary syndrome, pseudohypoparathyroidism, and insulinoma.[9] These potential causes are uncommon but should be considered as a part of the differential diagnosis. In each case, history, physical exam, and laboratory testing can be used to rule out these disorders.

Multiple autosomal-recessive defects have been described in association with human obesity. Dysmorphic mutations associated with human obesity include Prader-Willi, Cohen, Carpenter, Bardet-Biedl, and Alström syndromes.[9]

Medications occasionally are implicated in the genesis of obesity. These include phenothiazines, steroids, lithium, antiserotoninergic compounds, neuroleptics, and tricyclic antidepressants.[9]

Constructing a Treatment Plan[14–18]

Once a patient has been determined to be overweight or obese (having ruled out secondary causes), a treatment plan must be formulated. This should be discussed in detail with the patient. Obesity, especially in a society where beauty and thinness is held in high esteem, is difficult to manage and often accompanied with bouts of depression and extreme frustration for patients.[4] Depending on the staging of the patient, a nutritional consultation can be extremely important in getting off to a good start. The approach to management must be multilevel, and include detailed instruction and planning for exercise along with reduced-intake meal planning to create the necessary caloric deficit. In some instances, medications are useful either in the beginning of the treatment plan or as a continuous supplemental tool to maintain consistent progress to goal.

The family physician must probe for any emotional and psychological issues that serve to impede or contribute to blocking weight loss attempts. Personal family problems, marital dysfunction, and financial worries can be at the root of inconsistent weight management. Any significant social mores such as varied concepts of what constitutes beauty and idiosyncrasies common to specific populations should be taken into account in counseling. Obese patients are surprisingly frequently unaware of modifying factors in their lives that influence their success in losing weight.[17,18] These factors include personal health belief systems, such as believing extra weight is attractive to some persons; race; nutritional habits; and hair care issues, such as avoiding perspiration to protect chemical treatments.[15] If necessary, supportive psychotherapy or referral for counseling might be necessary, and should not be overlooked.

Exercise

Developing a pattern of routine exercise is one of the most difficult areas of change for the overweight patient. Many patients have lost or never had an appreciation of exercise for fun and energy production.[15,18] They instead envision the drudgery of work and depletion of their energy in association with exercising. Exercise then becomes an unpleasant task, and pleasure is not taken in the process. Long-term success is in many respects dependent on changing these erroneous concepts.[1,5,19] The patient who becomes "addicted" to an exercise regime invariably enjoys a better outcome even if weight loss goals are incompletely realized, due to improved self-esteem. Chronically overweight patients frequently overestimate the amount and quality of effective calorie burning exercise that they accomplish while underestimating the amount of food taken in.[15] This is a deadly self-deceit, which must be uncovered and brought into the patient's consciousness to increase the opportunity for success.[18] If the clinical history is not taken meticulously, the patient will continue believing misinformation about how much exercise is necessary for effective negative calorie balance.

A minimum of 4 or 5 days per week should be exercise days,[5,12] with each session lasting for at least 20 to 30 minutes. The patient's pulse should reach 60% to 80% of the age-specific target heart rate maximum as a goal.[14,15] Physicians should give overweight patients—in writing, on a prescription pad—an "exercise prescription," including suggested length of time for activities and the target pulse, which is calculated by subtracting their age from 220 and multiplying by 0.6 and 0.8 to get a range. Patient education charts and handouts with calorie-burning equivalents are very helpful to teach the concept of caloric deficit through increasing activity and decreasing intake. Encouraging incorporation of more walking, climbing stairs, and manual activities into daily routine is also beneficial.[1,14,16] It is critical for the patient to understand that temperature and weather changes must not deter efforts to maintain exercise. Many patients believe that pleasant weather is the only time to exercise.[15,18]

Food Intake

Many physicians refer patients for dietary counseling to determine and resolve the difficult problem of what and how much to eat. Another relatively simple approach that primary care physicians can incorporate into their practice is to determine by dietary history an estimate of the calories consumed daily, and then to assist the patient in diminishing 500 calories per day from that starting point.[5,16] This sets a goal of approximately a 3500-calorie deficit per week, leading minimally to a 1 pound per week weight loss calorie deficit. Many patients have difficulty in ascertaining exactly how much of each type of food on a percentage basis they should eat. Keeping daily total fat under 30% is a fair approximation of a more healthy diet. Generally the normal healthy diet has 30% to 35% fat, 15% protein, and about 50% carbohydrate (combined simple and complex). Measuring exact quantities of food often leads to "burn out" over the long haul. Changing habits by reducing excessive quantities of the wrong types of foods in large amounts frequently leads to better compliance.[15]

Medications

Overweight patients often inquire about the use of medications to enhance weight loss. These agents can be very helpful, but should not be considered the primary solution. Consider medications for patients who have a BMI >30, or for those with a BMI >27 and a condition such as arthritis, diabetes, or hypertension. Be aware of the contraindications. The following medications are currently thought to be useful as adjuncts for weight loss. The patient should be warned that behavioral and lifestyle changes must accompany any medications if success is to be realized. The development of tolerance to these medications is also very common, and physicians must be prepared with new plans and encouragement when plateaus are reached. In all cases, cessation of the drug has been shown to result in rapid reaccumulation of weight if lifestyle changes are not accomplished and maintained.[1,20]

Sibutramine (Meridia)

This drug suppresses appetite by blocking reuptake of norepinephrine and serotonin. Long-term safety is unknown. The medication has been associated with blood pressure elevation, dry mouth, insomnia, headache, and constipation. The usual dosage is 10 to 15 mg daily.[1,20] One approach is to try 10 mg for 60 days, and then 15 mg for another 60 days. If satisfactory weight loss is not achieved after this regime, the likelihood of success is very low.

Orlistat (Xenical)

Orlistat has been used safely in studies for up to 2 years. Patients have been found to lose weight with slow regain. Chemically, tetrahydrolipstatin is a lipase inhibitor and it decreases absorption of dietary fat. Use of this medication is contraindicated if the patient has a chronic malabsorption syndrome.[20] Adverse gastrointestinal effects are oily spotting, flatus, increased defecation, and fecal incontinence. The usual dose is 120 mg three times a day, taken with the three main meals.[1]

Phentermine (Adipex-P, Ionamin)

This medication stimulates release of norepinephrine and is given before meals to reduce appetite. The usual starting dose is 24 to 37.5 mg daily given either in divided doses or a single dose. Drugs from this group tend to produce more adverse effects than sibutramine.[20] These include dry mouth, gastrointestinal (GI) discomfort, nervousness, dizziness, hypertension, insomnia, tachycardia, agitated states, and libidinous changes.[1,20,21] This class of drugs also includes diethylpropion (Tenuate) and phendimetrazine (Bontril). Their contraindications and side effects are similar to those of phentermine.

Surgical Options

There is a place for surgical or bariatric treatment for obesity,[1] which should be reserved for patients who are clinically severely obese with a BMI ≥ 40 kg/m^2. Patients with a BMI >30 and one or more comorbid risk factors, such as diabetes, hypertension, arthritis, hyperlipidemia, or sleep apnea; and have been resistant to nonsurgical therapy are also considered candidates. Individuals who have made only minimal effort to lose weight by exercising and reducing intake should not be routinely referred for bariatric surgery for their convenience.

Currently, for those patients who appropriately qualify, the most successful procedures have been the Roux-en-Y gastric bypass or vertical banded gastroplasty procedures.[1] These surgeries have resulted in a 40% to 70% loss of excess body weight. The gastric bypass procedure is more effective than gastroplasty alone.[1] In experienced hands at most large medical centers, perioperative mortality is less than 1%. Many of these patients become independent of antihypertensive and diabetic medications. Improvements in the symptoms of degenerative arthritis can be anticipated. Risks include anastomotic leaks, wound infections, stomal stenosis, and incisional hernia.[1,14,16] Postoperative metabolic complications include vitamin and mineral deficiencies, especially iron and vitamin B$_{12}$. Some patients experience chronic nausea, vomiting, dumping syndrome, or constipation.[1]

Fad Diets

A fad diet is a weight loss scheme that touts a rapid result with very little effort. Many of these diets work for short periods of time, but usually have drawbacks of craving, nutritional inadequacy, or difficulty in maintenance. The successful diet always results in diminished overall total daily calories while simultaneously providing appropriate nutrients, vitamins, and minerals. Each diet should be analyzed individually for adequate amounts of protein, carbohydrate, fat, and fluid content. If necessary, seek a certified dietary consultation to evaluate diets or dietary supplements. Caution patients about the use of diets that include appetite-suppressant additives or over-the-counter food supplements, which could prove to be metabolically dangerous,[1,20,21] especially with comorbid conditions such as hypertension. Many of these supplements have caffeine, guarana, and or ma huang (ephedrine) to make the patient feel energetic about the program. There are no easy "fad" diet answers to the difficult problem of obesity.

Summary

Obesity is a serious chronic disease fraught with frustration, low self-esteem, multiple setbacks, and a poor prognosis for most patients.[5] Success must be measured individually, and patients must remain under continuous periodic medical attention to detect psychological, personal, and behavioral influences that can lead them back to previous bad habits. Restraint in eating, evaluation, therapy for emotional problems, continuous exercise, and lifestyle changes are the only interventions that can result in permanent weight loss.[9,11,21] In some cases personal and or genetic influences are so powerful that surgery is the only option left. Physicians treating these patients must take special care to remain encouraging and nonjudgmental in managing this tremendous medical problem that affects a large segment of society.

References

1. Obesity. June 2001. Available at *www.dynamicmedical.com.*
2. Kuczmarski RJ, Flegal KM, Campbell SM, et al. Increasing prevalence of overweight among US adults: The National Health and Nutrition Examination Survey, Phase 1, 1988–1991. JAMA 1994;272:205–11.

3. Flegal KM, Carroll MD, Kuczmarski RJ, et al. Overweight and obesity in the United States—prevalence and trends, 1960–1994. Int J Obes Relat Metab Disord 1998;22:39–47.
4. Martin LF, Hunter SM, Lauve RM, et al. Severe obesity: expensive to society, frustrating to treat, but important to confront. South Med J 1995;88:895–902.
5. Pi Sunyer FX. Medical hazards of obesity. Ann Intern Med 1993;119: 655–60.
6. Gibbs WW. Gaining on fat. Sci Am 1996;275:88–94.
7. Bray GA. Complications of obesity. Ann Intern Med 1985;103:1052–62.
8. McGinnis JM, Foege WH. Actual causes of death in the United States. JAMA 1993;270:2207–12.
9. Chan S, Blackburn GL. Helping patients reverse the health risks of obesity. J Clin Outc Manage 1997;4(3)37–50.
10. Wolf AM, Colditz GA. The cost of obesity: The U.S. Perspective. Pharmacoeconomics 1994;5(1 suppl):34–7.
11. Rippe JM, Yanovski SZ. Obesity—a chronic disease. Patient Care 1998;October 15:29–62.
12. NIH Consensus Statement, Physical Activity and Cardiovascular Health, vol 13, No. 3 Dec. 18–20, 1995.
13. Egger G. The case for using waist to hip ratio measurements in routine medical checks. Med J Aust 1992;156:280–5.
14. Guidance for treatment of adult obesity. Available at *www.shapeup.org*.
15. Railey MT. Evaluation and treatment of obesity. Prim Care Rep 1997;3(14):125–32.
16. Shikora SA, Saltzman E. Revisiting obesity: current treatment strategies. Hosp Med 1998;11:41–9.
17. Walcott-McQuigg JA, Sullivan J, Dan A, Logan B. Psychosocial factors influencing weight control behavior of African-American women. West J Nurs Res 1995;17:502–20.
18. Railey MT. Parameters of obesity in African-American Women. Nat Med Assoc 2000;92(10):481–4.
19. Report of the Secretary Task Force on Black and Minority Health. Executive summary, vol. 1, DHHS pub. 85-487367 (Q63). Washington, DC: U.S. Department of Health and Human Services, 1985.
20. Allison DB, Anderson JW, Aronne LJ, Campfield LA, Vash PD. Taking advantage of antiobesity medications. Patient Care 2000;11:34–62.
21. Agrawal M, Worzniak M, Diamond L. Managing obesity like any other chronic condition. Postgrad Med 2000;108(1):75–82.

5

Care of the Patient with Fatigue

John Saultz

Everyone experiences fatigue periodically as a result of hard physical labor or loss of sleep. Fatigue, loss of energy, and lassitude are also common symptoms experienced by patients with any of a large number of diseases. A patient who complains of fatigue presents a difficult problem for the family physician because there are many possible explanations for it. The subjective nature of the complaint and the potential seriousness of some of the diseases in the differential diagnosis compound this difficulty.

Background

Fatigue is common in the general population and is present in at least 20% of the patients who visit a family physician.[1–4] Community-based surveys indicate that as many as 50% of the population report fatigue if asked.[2,3] In the United States, fatigue is responsible for at least 10 million office visits and up to $300 million in health costs each year.[5] Valdini and colleagues[6] determined that 58% of family practice patients with a chief complaint of fatigue were still fatigued 1 year after the initial visit. But, in the absence of identifiable underlying organic diseases, 19 studies examining the prognosis of chronic fatigue found only three deaths among 2075 patients.[7] Chronic fatigue lasting over 6 months has a population prevalence of 1775/100,000 to 6321/100,000.[1] Fatigue consistently ranks among the most common presenting complaints to family physicians regardless of practice setting or culture. A systematic, organized, efficient evaluation of these patients represents an essential skill for all family physicians.

Although fatigue is common and often persistent, many chronically fatigued patients defy diagnostic categorization. For centuries physicians have been perplexed by the diagnostic difficulties inherent in evaluating patients with chronic fatigue. Clinical syndromes have been defined to explain chronic fatigue including terms such as febricula, neurasthenia, nervous exhaustion, Da Costa syndrome, chronic brucellosis, hypoglycemia, total allergy syndrome, chronic candidiasis, and chronic Epstein-Barr virus infection.[8] In 1987 the United States Centers for Disease Control (CDC) established a clinical definition for the chronic fatigue syndrome (CFS).[9] It was hoped that such categorization would facilitate clinical investigation of the causes and most successful treatments for this problem. But the case definition did not clearly identify a clinically useful subset of chronically fatigued patients, and the definition was revised in 1994.[10] This chapter reviews a contextual, biopsychosocial differential diagnosis of fatigue and outlines a practical approach to evaluating and helping patients who complain of fatigue

Clinical Presentation

What are the characteristics of patients who complain of fatigue to the family physician? There is a bimodal distribution of patient age, with a peak between the ages of 15 and 24 and a second peak at 60-plus years. Women complain of fatigue to the physician at least twice as often as men.[3–6,9,11,12] This excess may be explained by a higher incidence of fatigue in women, that women are more likely to tell the physician about fatigue, or that physicians are more sensitive to the ways in which women complain about fatigue. Fatigued patients tend to score lower than nonfatigued patients on tests that measure physical activity. They also score significantly higher than control patients on standardized instruments measuring anxiety and depression, and have a higher lifetime likelihood of being diagnosed with these disorders.[5,13,14]

It is useful to consider the clinical presentation of fatigue in different contexts depending on how the patient describes the problem. Some patients experience fatigue as part of a larger symptom complex in which the fatigue is identified only on detailed history or review of systems by the physician. Other patients present with a chief complaint of fatigue. A third group of patients presents to the physician specifically with questions about CFS. Patients rarely report acute fatigue to the physician when they have an understanding of why the fatigue is present. For example, a patient who is experiencing a common viral illness usually expects fatigue to be part of the symptom complex and is less likely to be concerned enough to complain about fatigue to the physician. Such patients would not present to the family physician complaining of fatigue but would admit to fatigue on a review of systems. Thus fatigue is a secondary symptom to these patients.

Most studies that have addressed fatigue in family practice have examined only those patients in whom fatigue was the chief or primary complaint. Such a complaint generally causes the physician to consider a long differential diagnosis of diseases that may cause fatigue as a primary symptom. In this clinical situation, the ability to address a broad differential diagnosis in a cost-efficient manner is essential. CFS has received substantial publicity in the lay press. For this reason, a number of patients present to the family physician with questions about this disorder. It is important for the family physician to understand the diagnostic criteria of CFS and to be familiar with the latest research in this area.

Diagnosis

Few patient problems illustrate the inadequacies of the biomedical model of diagnosis more clearly than does fatigue. A diagnostic model that examines the patient's complaint and attempts to determine its cause and then apply a treatment regimen to that cause is called an "epidemiologic model." The traditional biomedical model of diagnosis is largely an epidemiologic model. A contextual model of diagnosis, instead of attempting to identify cause, attempts to identify associated symptoms and factors that make the patient's complaint easier to understand and manage.[15] Contextual diagnosis can include a biomedical approach to the patient but necessarily also includes family, community, and sociocultural considerations. What follows is a contextual approach to diagnosis when a patient complains of fatigue as a secondary concern or chief complaint, or has concerns about CFS.

Fatigue as a Secondary Symptom

Many of the most common problems seen by family physicians are problems associated with fatigue. Chronic medical conditions such as diabetes, commonly prescribed medications such as antihypertensives, acute illnesses such as viral hepatitis, physiologic changes such as pregnancy, and stressful life situations such as divorce may be associated with fatigue. In these situations, fatigue often is identified as a secondary symptom and, from a diagnostic point of view, may be relatively unimportant. From a contextual point of view, however, the family physician is interested in the degree to which the patient's fatigue is interfering with job performance, family relationships, physical activity, or sexual activity. The contextual approach requires the physician to be as interested in the effects of symptoms as in their cause. Thus when fatigue is a secondary symptom, its importance may rest with its effect on the patient's lifestyle and coping skills for the underlying illness.

Fatigue as a Presenting Complaint

Few clinical situations more fully exercise the skills of a family physician than the patient who presents with a chief complaint of unexplained fatigue. Table 5.1 lists some of the medical and psychosocial problems associated with a chief complaint of fatigue. Evaluation of such a patient begins with a careful, comprehensive medical history, which includes a detailed psychosocial history including symptoms of depression, sleep disorders, anxiety disorders, substance abuse, and the marital and sexual experience.

The most common causes of fatigue as a presenting complaint to a family physician are depression, life stress, chronic medical illnesses, and medication reactions. The history must also include information about the other symptoms of such illnesses as those listed in Table 5.1.

The complete medical history is followed by a careful physical examination. Areas of particular importance on the physical examination are the thyroid gland, cardiovascular system, rectum, pelvis, and mental status (for associated signs of depression or anxiety disorders).

Laboratory evaluation of the patient who presents with chronic fatigue, though important to consider, is unlikely to be helpful in most cases. Sugarman and Berg[16] found that laboratory testing was helpful in securing a diagnosis in only nine of 118 fatigued patients in a university family practice clinic. An appropriate laboratory evaluation is directed by the history and physical examination. For most patients, testing includes a complete blood count, a serum chemistry profile, an erythrocyte sedimentation rate (as a screen for inflammatory disorders), and thyroid-stimulating hormone level (as a screen for hypothyroidism). Other laboratory tests, including a chest radio-

Table 5.1. **Diagnoses Associated with Fatigue**

Infectious diseases	**Vascular disorders**
Viral syndromes	Atherosclerotic heart disease
Mononucleosis	Valvular heart disease
Hepatitis	Congestive heart failure
Pharyngitis	Cardiomyopathy
Endocarditis	Congenital heart disorders
Urinary tract infections	
HIV infection	**Pulmonary conditions**
Tuberculosis	Asthma/COPD
	Allergic disorders
Toxins and drug effects	Restrictive lung diseases
Medication side effects	
Alcohol and drug abuse	**Miscellaneous conditions**
Chronic poisoning	Anemia
	Pregnancy
Endocrine and metabolic problems	Systemic lupus erythematosus
	Iron deficiency
Electrolyte disturbance	Renal failure
Hypothyroidism	Chronic liver disease
Hypoglycemia	Multiple sclerosis
Diabetes	Sleep disorders including sleep apnea
Hyperthyroidism	
Starvation or dieting	**Psychosocial problems**
Obesity	Depression
Adrenal insufficiency	Anxiety disorders
	Adjustment reaction
Neoplastic conditions	Situational life stress
Occult malignancy	Alcohol and drug abuse
Leukemia and lymphoma	Sexual dysfunction
Carcinoma of the colon	Spouse abuse, child abuse, or other family violence
	Occupational stress and professional burnout syndrome

HIV = human immunodeficiency virus; COPD = chronic obstructive pulmonary disease.

graph, electrocardiogram, urinalysis, and tuberculin skin testing, may be indicated, depending on the results of the history and physical examination.

Patients without a readily apparent explanation for their fatigue should also be evaluated with a careful family assessment. Such an assessment may include convening a family meeting, preparing a family genogram, or using other family assessment instruments. An assessment of the occupational history, living environment, and social and financial circumstances should also be included in the complete evaluation of patients with fatigue.

Chronic Fatigue Syndrome

The CDC's definition of CFS is outlined in Table 5.2.[10] The purpose of establishing these diagnostic criteria was to identify a subgroup of fatigued patients to direct future research studies. Research projects have since focused on learning more about patients who meet these criteria. Because of obvious similarities to infectious mononucleosis, a number of studies have searched for an association with viral infections. Although these investigations continue, there is no good evidence to link CFS and viral infections.[17–20] Other research has examined the immune function of patients with CFS. Although measurable immune abnormalities have been associated with CFS, no consistent pattern has been delineated from study to study.[17,19,20] Another area of ongoing research has been an attempt to associate connective tissue and autoimmune diseases with CFS. Only a few patients have abnormal autoantibodies, and no association with autoimmune diseases has been clearly established.[21] More recent studies have examined the hypothesis that abnormalities of the central nervous system or changes in the regulation of the hypothalamic-pituitary-adrenal axis might explain chronic fatigue. At this time, evidence of a clinically useful association is inconclusive.[18,19,22,23] Finally, studies have examined the relationship between chronic fatigue and psychiatric disorders. These studies suggest that depression alone is insufficient to explain most cases of chronic or persistent fatigue.[19,22] Several recent studies have raised questions about the degree of diagnostic overlap between chronic fatigue and other conditions such as fibromyalgia and irritable bowel syndrome. Clinically important fatigue is present in over 75% of patients with fibromyalgia and many patients with chronic fatigue have demonstrable trigger points on musculoskeletal exam. Some authors suggest that the family of functional somatic syndromes may in fact be different manifestations of the same process.[24–26] It now seems clear that patients with CFS are not a homogeneous group and are not different from other patients with chronic fatigue in most respects.

It is also clear that chronic fatigue is much more common than CFS. Fewer than 5% of patients who present with chronic fatigue to a family physician ultimately fulfill the diagnostic criteria for CFS.[1,11] Patients who present to the family physician concerned about CFS represent a complex challenge. Some patients are simply looking for information, a need that can be met by discussing questions and providing educational resources. Many patients who are concerned about CFS do not satisfy the criteria listed in Table 5.2 sufficiently to qualify for this diagnosis. These patients require a contextual diagnostic approach from the physician.

Table 5.2. **Case Definition: Chronic Fatigue Syndrome and Idiopathic Chronic Fatigue**

Prolonged fatigue is self-reported, persistent fatigue lasting 1 month or longer. Chronic fatigue is self-reported persistent or relapsing fatigue lasting 6 or more consecutive months.

A case of *chronic fatigue syndrome* is defined as chronic fatigue that is not explained by medical conditions that adequately explain the fatigue (see below) with the presence of the following:

1. clinically evaluated, unexplained, persistent or relapsing chronic fatigue that is of new or definite onset, is not the result of ongoing exertion, is not substantially relieved by rest, and results in substantial reduction in previous levels of occupational, educational, social, or personal activities; and
2. the concurrent occurrence of four or more of the following symptoms, all of which must have persisted or recurred during 6 or more consecutive months and must not have predated the fatigue:

   self-reported impairment in short-term memory or concentration severe enough to cause substantial reduction in previous levels of occupational, educational, social, or personal activities
   sore throat
   tender cervical or axillary lymph nodes
   muscle pain
   multijoint pain without joint swelling or redness
   headaches of a new type, pattern, or severity
   unrefreshing sleep
   postexertional malaise lasting more than 24 hours

A case of *idiopathic chronic fatigue* is defined as clinically evaluated, unexplained chronic fatigue that fails to meet the criteria for chronic fatigue syndrome.

The following conditions exclude the patient from being classified as unexplained chronic fatigue:

   Any active medical condition that may explain chronic fatigue including medication side effects
   Any previously diagnosed medical condition whose resolution has not been documented beyond a reasonable doubt and whose continued activity may explain chronic fatigue
   Any past or current diagnosis of a major depressive disorder with psychotic or melancholic features, bipolar affective disorder, schizophrenia of any subtype, delusional disorders of any subtype, dementias of any subtype, or bulimia nervosa
   Alcohol or substance abuse within 2 years before the onset of chronic fatigue or at any time afterward
   Severe obesity defined as a body mass index equal to or greater than 45

(continued)

Table 5.2 (Continued).

The following conditions do not exclude the patient from being classified as unexplained chronic fatigue:

  Any condition defined primarily by symptoms that cannot be confirmed by diagnostic laboratory tests, including fibromyalgia, anxiety disorders, somatoform disorders, nonpsychotic or nonmelancholic depression, neurasthenia, and multiple chemical sensitivity disorder

  Any condition under specific treatment sufficient to alleviate all symptoms related to that condition and for which the adequacy of treatment has been documented

  Any condition, such as Lyme disease or syphilis, that was treated with definitive therapy before development of symptomatic sequelae

  Any isolated and explained physical examination finding or laboratory or imagining test abnormality that is insufficient to strongly suggest the existence of an exclusionary condition

Evaluation of the chronic fatigue patient should begin with a comprehensive history and physical examination. Most patients have previously seen other physicians for this problem, and copies of previous medical records from these physicians should be obtained. At the initial visit it is imperative that the physician discuss in detail the way in which chronic fatigue has affected and changed the patient's life. A careful family assessment should be completed, including convening the family whenever possible. Although chronic fatigue patients have a high prevalence of depression, anxiety disorders, somatization disorders, and family dysfunction, patients may not be receptive to discussing psychosocial issues early in the process of caring for this problem. Because biomedical evaluation is unlikely to yield a definitive diagnosis, a complete biopsychosocial evaluation beginning at the initial visit is crucial. Patients should be seen frequently, and the laboratory evaluation should include those studies described above for the patient with a chief complaint of chronic fatigue. At the present time there is little justification for extensive immunologic or autoimmune diagnostic testing. Focused laboratory tests should be ordered when indicated from the history and physical examination.

Management

In an epidemiologic model, management of the problem begins after the correct diagnosis has been determined. With a contextual approach, management begins at the time of initial contact between the patient and physician. Caring for patients with a primary complaint of fatigue requires a contextual approach, which means that the physician's diagnostic inquiry must include the broadest possible scope. The physician begins at the initial visit to assist the patient in delineating ways to cope with the symptoms more effectively. What follows are the basic principles of a systemic management plan for a patient with a primary complaint of chronic fatigue.

1. The physician must be as interested and concerned about the effects of the patient's fatigue as about its cause. Delineating the effects of the symptom on the patient's life is an important step in understanding the symptom and managing the problem.
2. The physician should explain to the patient at the initial visit that the most common causes of fatigue as a presenting complaint are depression and psychosocial problems. The physician should ascertain what this information means to the patient and whether the patient thinks that psychosocial issues may play a role in the fatigue.
3. The physician should discuss the other common causes of fatigue with the patient at the initial visit and ask the patient to think about these possibilities between the initial and first follow-up visit. At the first follow-up visit the physician can then inquire as to whether the patient has had an opportunity to consider possible explanations for the fatigue and if there is new insight into the problem.
4. The physician should continue to return to the discussion of family, occupational, psychosexual, and substance abuse issues at each of the follow-up visits. This can take place while a detailed biomedical evaluation of the patient's symptoms is progressing. Even if fatigue is being caused by a physical disorder, there are important effects on family and job.
5. The physician can consider convening the family to explore the attitudes and ideas of other family members. This point is especially important if the patient has a spouse or significant other.
6. The physician should be able to discuss professional burnout, career dissatisfaction, and other issues that are outside the usual biomedical model of thinking about patient problems. It may be helpful to provide patients with copies of articles about fatigue. Some studies suggest that cognitive-behavioral therapy may be beneficial for patients with chronic fatigue.[27]
7. If the physician believes that a psychosocial problem is of primary importance to the patient's condition but the patient is un-

willing to accept this explanation, the biomedical workup should be paced slowly and scheduled across several follow-up visits. This will allow the doctor–patient rapport to deepen and discussions about psychosocial concerns to continue.

8. The physician should refer the patient to a consultant only for a well-specified purpose. It is essential to communicate with consultants in advance and to avoid using consultants who lack sophistication about psychosocial issues.

9. Prolonged rest is more likely to harm than help patients with chronic fatigue. A gradual program of activity has resulted in improved functional status in some studies.

10. Tricyclic or selective serotonin reuptake inhibitor antidepressants may benefit some patients, particularly those with disturbed sleep patterns. When used, these medications should be started in low doses and their therapeutic effect should be carefully monitored.[28,29]

Summary

Acute fatigue may be a presenting complaint for a large number of important diseases. Fatigue has a large biomedical differential diagnosis and requires a broad contextual approach to optimize diagnosis and management. Although few presenting complaints are more challenging, few patient problems more urgently require the broad contextual diagnostic approach that can best be provided by the family physician.

References

1. Buchwald D, Umali P, Umali J, Kith P, Pearlman T, Komaroff AL. Chronic fatigue and the chronic fatigue syndrome: prevalence in a Pacific Northwest health care system. Ann Intern Med 1995;123:81–8.

2. Kroenke K, Wood DR, Mangelsdorff D, Meier NJ, Powell JB. Chronic fatigue in primary care. JAMA 1988;260:929–34.

3. Pawlikowska T, Chalder T, Hirsch SR, et al. Population based study of fatigue and psychological distress. BMJ 1994;308:763–6.

4. Shahar E, Lederer J. Asthenic symptoms in a rural family practice. J Fam Pract 1990;31:257–62.

5. Kirk J, Douglass R, Nelson E, et al. Chief complaint of fatigue: a prospective study. J Fam Pract 1990;30:33–41.

6. Valdini AF, Steinhardt S, Valicenti J, Jaffe A. A one-year follow-up of fatigued patients. J Fam Pract 1988;26:33–8.

7. Joyce J, Hotopf M, Wessely S. The prognosis of chronic fatigue and chronic fatigue syndrome: a systematic review. Q J Med 1997;90: 223–33.

8. Straus SE. History of chronic fatigue syndrome. Rev Infect Dis 1991; 13(suppl 1):S2–S7.

9. Holmes GP, Kaplan JE, Gantz NM, et al. Chronic fatigue syndrome: a working case definition. Ann Intern Med 1988;108:387–9.

10. Fukuda K, Straus SE, Hickie I, Sharpe M, Dobbins JG, Komaroff AL. The chronic fatigue syndrome: a comprehensive approach to its definition and study. Ann Intern Med 1994;121:953–9.

11. Manu P, Lane TJ, Matthews DA. The frequency of the chronic fatigue syndrome in patients with symptoms of persistent fatigue. Ann Intern Med 1988;109:554–6.

12. Morrison JD. Fatigue as a presenting complaint in family practice. J Fam Pract 1980;10:795–801.

13. Cathebras PJ, Robbins JM, Kirmayer LJ, Hayton BC. Fatigue in primary care: prevalence, psychiatric comorbidity, illness behavior, and outcome. J Gen Intern Med 1992;7:276–86.

14. Kroenke K, Spitzer RL, Williams JB, et al. Physical symptoms in primary care. Predictors of psychiatric disorders and functional impairment. Arch Fam Med 1994;3:774–9.

15. Saultz JW. Contextual care. In: Saultz JW, ed. Textbook of family medicine. New York: McGraw-Hill, 2000;135–59.

16. Sugarman JR, Berg AD. Evaluation of fatigue in a family practice. J Fam Pract 1984;19:643–7.

17. Glaser R, Kiecolt-Glaser JK. Stress-associated immune modulation: relevance to viral infections and chronic fatigue syndrome. Am J Med 1998;105:35S–42S.

18. Johnson SK, DeLuca J, Natelson BH. Chronic fatigue syndrome: reviewing the research findings. Ann Behav Med 1999;21:258–71.

19. Komaroff AL, Buchwald DS. Chronic fatigue syndrome: an update. Annu Rev Med 1998;49:1–13.

20. Mawle AC. Chronic fatigue syndrome. Immunol Invest 1997;26:269–73.

21. Buchwald DS, Komaroff AL. Review of laboratory findings for patients with chronic fatigue syndrome. Rev Infect Dis 1991;13(suppl 1): S12–S18.

22. Demitrack MA. Chronic fatigue syndrome and fibromyalgia. Dilemmas in diagnosis and clinical management. Psychiatr Clin North Am 1998;21:671–92.

23. Demitrack MA, Crofford LJ. Evidence for and pathophysiologic implications of hypothalamic-pituitary-adrenal axis dysregulation in fibromyalgia and chronic fatigue syndrome. Ann NY Acad Sci 1998;840: 684–97.

24. Bennett R. Fibromyalgia, chronic fatigue syndrome, and myofascial pain. Curr Opin Rheumatol 1998;10:95–103.

25. Goldenberg DL. Fibromyalgia, chronic fatigue syndrome, and myofascial pain syndrome. Curr Opin Rheumatol 1997;9:135–43.

26. Wessely S, Nimnuan C, Sharpe M. Functional somatic syndromes: one or many? Lancet 1999;354:936–9.

27. Butler S, Chalder T, Ron M, Wessely S. Cognitive behaviour therapy in chronic fatigue syndrome. J Neurol Neurosurg Psychiatry 1991;54: 153–8.

28. Brunello N, Akiskal H, Boyer P, et al. Dysthymia: clinical picture, extent of overlap with chronic fatigue syndrome, neuropharmacological considerations, and new therapeutic vistas. J Affect Disord 1999;52: 275–90.

29. O'Malley PG, Jackson JL, Santoro J, Tomkins G, Balden E, Kroenke K. Antidepressant therapy for unexplained symptoms and symptom syndromes. J Fam Pract 1999;48:980–90.

6
Care of the Patient with a Sleep Disorder

Thomas A. Johnson, Jr.
and James J. Deckert

Sleep is a periodically recurring physiologic state of lessened responsiveness from which one can be readily awakened. The quality and quantity of sleep vary with age. Newborns sleep an average of 16 hours each day in randomly fragmented fashion. As an individual matures, sleep usually coalesces into a single prolonged nighttime period, with an average length of 7 to 8 hours in adults. A few individuals function well with as little as 4 hours per day, whereas others require 10 hours or more.

Sleep architecture also evolves with age. Slow wave sleep (SWS), the stage of deepest sleep, is maximal in young children and decreases gradually through midlife.[1] Older adults often take longer to fall asleep, take daytime naps, and experience more frequent awakenings. A wide variety of disorders can interfere with normal sleep patterns.

Insomnia

Insomnia can be clinically defined as any difficulty falling or staying asleep that results in impaired daytime functioning. Inadequate sleep can result in fatigue, decreased concentration, and irritability. Insomnia can be classified as acute or chronic.

Acute insomnia is difficulty sleeping that lasts 1 month or less. The cause is generally some situational stress readily identified or even anticipated by the patient. Examinations, funerals, vacations, and illnesses are examples of stresses that frequently precipitate acute insomnia. Patients often tolerate this brief disruption without bringing it to the attention of their physician.

In contrast, chronic insomnia is a significant health problem, often frustrating to patients and their physicians. The etiology is often multifactorial. Underlying causes cover a spectrum of behavioral, psychiatric, and medical disorders (Table 6.1). It is essential that the physician clarify, as much as possible, the cause of insomnia before attempting treatment.

Table 6.1. **Causes of Insomnia**

Drug-induced insomnia
Nonprescription: alcohol, decongestants, caffeine, nicotine (smoking)
Prescription: amphetamines, stimulating tricyclics, thyroid hormones, β-agonists, aminophyllines, beta-blockers, steroids, diuretics, sedatives (withdrawal), serotonin reuptake inhibitors, oral contraceptives

Psychiatric disease
Affective disorders: depression, bipolar disorder, dysthymic disorders
Anxiety disorders: generalized anxiety disorders, panic disorder, posttraumatic stress
Schizophrenia

Medical problems
Gastrointestinal: reflux esophagitis, peptic ulcer disease, inflammatory bowel disease
Cardiac: angina, paroxysmal nocturnal dyspnea
Genitourinary: pregnancy, urinary tract infection, benign prostatic hypertrophy, uremia
Respiratory: chronic obstructive pulmonary disease, asthma
Endocrine: hyperthyroidism, diabetes, Cushing syndrome, Addison syndrome, menopause
Skin: pruritus
Central nervous system: dementia, delirium, seizure disorder
Musculoskeletal: arthritis, fibromyalgia
Pain from any source

Primary sleep disorders
Poor sleep hygiene
Primary insomnia
Circadian rhythm disturbance
Sleep apnea
Periodic limb movements and restless legs syndrome

Evaluation

Patients often seek physician advice regarding insomnia. However, more than half of patients with concerns about sleep fail to discuss the problem with their doctor.[2] Incorporating a brief sleep history into the review of systems is helpful in detecting these individuals. If the history is consistent with chronic insomnia, the following areas need to be explored.

Drugs

A review of the patient's drug use is essential. Alcohol, often self-prescribed to induce sleep, can produce abnormal sleep architecture and early awakening. Caffeine has a long half-life (8–14 hours) and can interfere with sleep onset long after consumption. Nicotine, through smoking or administered as a drug, can produce enough arousal to interfere with sleep initiation. A variety of over-the-counter and prescription drugs can cause insomnia (Table 6.1). If discontinuation of the offending medication is not feasible, a change in the timing of administration may be helpful.

Psychiatric Disorders

Psychiatric disorders, particularly depression and anxiety, are common causes of sleep disturbance. Screening questions for these disorders can generally uncover the diagnosis. Referral to a psychiatrist is sometimes appropriate if more severe psychiatric disorder, such as schizophrenia, is suspected.

Medical Disorders

A variety of medical problems can cause insomnia (Table 6.1). Occult medical problems are a particularly common etiology of sleep disruption in the elderly. A complete history, physical exam, and appropriate laboratory testing should be conducted to rule out suspected medical causes.

Primary Sleep Disorders

Poor sleep hygiene frequently contributes to insomnia, but it is seldom the sole cause. The rules of good sleep hygiene are listed in Table 6.2. Patients can initially be evaluated by history, but a more accurate assessment is obtained by utilizing a sleep diary to record details of the sleep pattern over a period of 1 to 2 weeks.

Circadian rhythm disturbance is also common. Patients whose jobs require shift work or excessive plane travel are often unable to

Table 6.2. **Rules of Good Sleep Hygiene**

Maintain regular bedtime and time of arising.

Avoid naps.

Exercise regularly, but avoid exercise just prior to bedtime.

Control sleep environment to avoid temperature extremes and
excessive noise.

Provide for a wind-down time of at least 30 minutes of non-stressful
activities prior to bedtime.

Reserve the bedroom for sleep and sexual activity only, eliminating
stimulating activities such as watching television, reading, paying
bills, making phone calls.

Go to bed only when ready for sleep and leave if unable to sleep
after 30 minutes.

fall asleep on schedule. These individuals should be questioned regarding drug use, as they often aggravate their sleep disturbance by excessive use of caffeine, nicotine, alcohol, and sedatives. Another type of circadian rhythm disturbance is delayed sleep-phase syndrome. This syndrome consists of early night insomnia with chronically late bedtimes and arising times. Delayed sleep-phase syndrome is particularly common in adolescents. In contrast, older individuals often complain of early morning waking with a tendency to fall asleep too early in the evening. This is designated advanced sleep-phase syndrome. Jet lag, perhaps the most common circadian rhythm disturbance.

Finally, primary insomnia is the diagnosis of exclusion and should be reserved for patients in whom known secondary causes have been ruled out or treated.

Treatment

The easiest, most effective treatment for insomnia is specific to an identified cause. A change in drug use or treatment of an underlying psychiatric/medical disorder often results in a dramatic improvement in sleep pattern. Nonspecific treatment for primary insomnia is generally less effective.

Nonpharmacologic Measures

A number of nonpharmacologic interventions have been found helpful in treating insomnia. These interventions include sleep hygiene education, cognitive therapy, sleep restriction, relaxation techniques, and light therapy.

Sleep Hygiene Education. Education regarding the rules of good sleep hygiene (Table 6.2) is helpful for most patients with insomnia. A sleep diary is valuable for identifying needed improvements and monitoring progress. The physician can help the patient select changes and can provide follow-up to encourage compliance.

Cognitive-Behavioral Therapy. Cognitive-behavioral therapy is a training program designed to correct misconceptions about sleep that may be adversely affecting a patient's sleep pattern. In some individuals, for example, concerns about amount of sleep needed or exaggerated fears about the effect of insomnia may generate excessive anxiety. This anxiety, in turn, interferes with their ability to initiate and maintain sleep. The goal of therapy is to diminish the anxiety surrounding sleep by changing the patient's understanding and attitude about the problem.[3]

Sleep Restriction Therapy. Sleep restriction therapy is a technique used to improve sleep efficiency. This approach is most useful for patients who spend an excessive amount of sleepless time in bed. Patients are instructed to limit the amount of time they spend in bed to the average amount of time they actually spend sleeping based on their sleep diary. Initially this practice results in some degree of sleep deprivation, but it helps to consolidate the sleep pattern. The patient is then instructed to gradually increase time in bed while maintaining sleep efficiency at more than 85% (i.e., more than 85% of time in bed is spent sleeping).

Relaxation Techniques. A wide variety of relaxation techniques may be useful for treating insomnia. Common approaches include progressive muscle relaxation, abdominal breathing, meditation, self-hypnosis, biofeedback, and imagery. All of these techniques are about equally effective, so choice is based on the therapist's experience and patient preference. Relaxation works best in patients with primary insomnia and those with associated anxiety disorders. Referral to a behaviorist is generally required unless the physician is skilled in teaching these techniques.

Light Therapy. Light therapy consists of exposing patients to bright light to manipulate their biologic clock. Exposure during the evening tends to cause a phase delay (i.e., delays sleep onset), whereas early morning exposure causes a phase advance (i.e., promotes earlier sleep onset). Light therapy is most useful for circadian rhythm disturbances.

Pharmacologic Therapy

Prescription Drugs. Hypnotic drugs are clearly useful for the treatment of transient insomnia. Prescribing a short-acting hypnotic can minimize sleep disruption during a stressful period and improve daytime functioning.

The role of hypnotics in chronic insomnia is more controversial. Although hypnotics are widely used for these patients, most published guidelines caution against using drugs in this setting. If a drug is prescribed for chronic insomnia, it should be prescribed in the lowest effective dose to minimize side effects. Recent studies suggest intermittent use of a short-acting hypnotic (i.e., 3 to 5 nights per week) may be the safest, most efficacious approach.[4,5]

The most commonly used hypnotics are the benzodiazepines and benzodiazepine receptor agonists (Table 6.3). The critical difference among these drugs is their duration of action. Short-acting drugs such as zolpidem (Ambien) produce minimal daytime sedation, but they are more likely to result in early awakening. Conversely, long-acting drugs such as flurazepam (Dalmane) reliably produce a full night's sleep at the cost of increased daytime drowsiness and potential accumulation effects.[6]

The newest hypnotic available in this class is zaleplon (Sonata). This drug is a pyrazolopyrimidine that binds selectively to benzodiazepine receptors. Zaleplon (Sonata) has an extremely short half-life, resulting in a duration of action of approximately 4 hours.[6] This brief duration of action allows PRN administration during the night, after the patient has experienced difficulty falling asleep.

The choice of hypnotic depends on the patient's specific needs. Individuals who have difficulty initiating sleep would be good candidates for a short-acting drug. Patients with symptoms of daytime anxiety or early awakening may do better with an intermediate- or long-acting drug.

Table 6.3. **Selected Hypnotics**

Drug	Duration of action	Half-life (hours)	Usual daily dosage (mg)
Zaleplon (Sonata)	Ultra-short	1	5–10
Zolpidem (Ambien)	Short	2.4	5–10
Triazolam (Halcion)	Short	1.5–5.5	0.125–0.250
Estazolam (ProSom)	Intermediate	10–24	1–2
Temazepam (Restoril)	Intermediate	8–10	15–30
Flurazepam (Dalmane)	Long	47–100	15–30
Quazepam (Doral)	Long	39	7.5–15.0

A number of older prescription hypnotics such as barbiturates, chloral hydrate, and meprobamate are still available. These drugs are not recommended due to their relatively high toxicity and the increased risk of dependence.[6]

Some patients are not good candidates for hypnotic drugs. These drugs are relatively contraindicated in patients with known drug abuse potential, including those with a history of alcohol dependence. Patients taking other central nervous system (CNS) depressants, such as pain relievers or antidepressants, should be dosed carefully with an awareness of possible drug potentiation. Hypnotics should be avoided if sleep apnea is suspected. Pregnancy is a contraindication owing to possible effects on the fetus. Individuals who must function well when awakened during the night (e.g., physicians, firemen) should be warned of possible impairment. Finally, hypnotics must be used with caution in the elderly. Older patients are more likely to exhibit side effects, such as confusion, amnesia, and dizziness. They are also at risk for secondary complications including hip fracture.[7] Because of age-related prolongation of half-life, long-acting drugs are more likely to accumulate to toxic levels and should seldom be used in this age group.

Sedating antidepressants are often prescribed for insomnia. Trazodone (Desyrel) in doses of 25 to 150 mg at bedtime is widely used. However, in the nondepressed patient, there is little data to support this approach. The clearest indications for treating insomnia with antidepressants are in patients with underlying depression or in those with a history of substance abuse.

Nonprescription Drugs. Two antihistamines are currently approved and marketed as "sleep-aids": diphenhydramine (Nytol) and doxylamine (Unisom). These drugs are long acting and only modestly effective. They can produce daytime drowsiness, impair performance, and have a high incidence of anticholinergic side effects such as dry mouth and urinary retention.

Melatonin is an over-the-counter hormone preparation that has attracted considerable public attention for its proposed hypnotic properties. Although secreted by the pineal gland during nighttime hours, it is not clear that melatonin supplementation induces or maintains sleep. There are few controlled studies, the therapeutic results are mixed, and long-term safety has not been established. The most convincing trials have demonstrated efficacy in blind patients and others with circadian rhythm disturbances.[8] Despite its possible benefits and apparent short-term safety, melatonin probably should not be recommended to most patients until better studies are conducted.

Herbal therapy is increasingly used by those seeking "natural" alternatives. Valerian root, kava, chamomile, passionflower, lemon balm, and lavender are among the herbal options marketed for insomnia. Of these, valerian root is the best studied and is mildly effective in bedtime doses of 200 to 900 mg. However, as with most herbal products, the optimal dose is uncertain and purity/safety is a major concern.

Narcolepsy

Narcolepsy is a relatively uncommon sleep disorder that typically presents in adolescence or early adulthood. The illness is characterized by excessive daytime sleepiness with a tendency to fall asleep uncontrollably even during stimulating activities. These irresistible sleep episodes generally last 10 to 30 minutes and sometimes occur suddenly, without warning. This sudden onset can put the patient at risk while participating in dangerous activities such as working or driving. The other major symptom of narcolepsy is cataplexy. Cataplexy occurs in about two thirds of patients with narcolepsy and consists of a sudden loss of muscle tone precipitated by an emotion such as laughter or surprise. When present, cataplexy is considered pathognomonic for the disorder. Other associated symptoms can include sleep paralysis and hypnagogic hallucinations.

Evaluation of patients suspected of having narcolepsy is complex and generally requires referral to a sleep laboratory. This evaluation, which should include a multiple sleep latency test (MSLT), can frequently confirm the diagnosis. Confirmation is important, as treatment includes potent CNS stimulants with addictive potential and black-market value. Narcolepsy is sometimes feigned to obtain these drugs.

Behavioral therapy consists chiefly of optimizing sleep hygiene and scheduling daytime naps. Drug therapy focuses on administration of stimulants for control of daytime sleepiness. Stimulants typically used include methylphenidate (Ritalin), dextroamphetamine (Dexedrine), and modafinil (Provigil).[9] Cataplexy may respond to antidepressants, including tricyclics and selective serotonin reuptake inhibitors (SSRIs).

Sleep Apnea

Sleep apnea consists of repeated episodes of complete (apnea) or partial (hypopnea) pharyngeal obstructions during sleep. These physiologic events plus the symptom of daytime somnolence characterize the obstructive sleep apnea syndrome (OSAS). This important syndrome is common, dangerous, and underdiagnosed. Approximately 2% to 4% of middle-aged adults have OSAS.[10] Sleep apnea is typically a disease of middle age and beyond. Also children can develop sleep apnea, typically from adenotonsillar hypertrophy. Although pregnant women often snore, overt OSAS is uncommon.

The recurrent arousals and associated episodes of transient hypertension followed the next day by daytime somnolence of OSAS often results in significant increased risk of traffic accidents, poor job and social performance, as well as cardiovascular and cerebrovascular disease. There is a 37% death rate over 8 years of diagnosis seen in untreated OSAS.[11]

There is significant overlap between hypertension and sleep apnea. Approximately 30% of middle-aged men with primary hypertension have OSAS, and more than 40% of patients with OSAS have daytime hypertension. Also, the treatment of OSAS frequently reduces daytime systemic blood pressure.[12] It is, therefore, important to inquire about sleep apnea symptoms in patients with hypertension.

Diagnosis

Apnea is defined as cessation of airflow for at least 10 seconds. This is typically associated with what is called sleep fragmentation as measured by electroencephalographic (EEG) arousal during an overnight polysomnogram and a 2% to 4% decline in oxygen saturation during the apneic episode. An hypopnea is a reduction in airflow that results in an arousal and/or oxygen desaturation.

An overnight polysomnographic study is the best way to diagnose this syndrome. It should be performed for (1) patients who habitually snore and report daytime sleepiness and (2) those who habitually snore and have observed apnea (regardless of daytime symptoms). Snoring is generally the first symptom of sleep apnea. It is produced by vibration of soft tissues within the upper airway. The polysomnogram report will include a measure of the respiratory disturbance index (RDI), which is the number of abnormal breathing events per hour of sleep.

The characteristic nocturnal symptom pattern is loud snoring or brief gasps that alternate with 20 to 30 seconds of silence. These apnea events are noted by 75% of bed partners. Snoring intensity increases with weight gain and sedative or heavy alcohol intake, all of which lead to flaccidity of the pharyngeal tissues. Also, the pharyngeal trauma resulting from the repeated vibrations of untreated OSAS causes further pharyngeal changes, resulting in worsening of the syndrome in that patient. Half of patients toss and turn at night. About a quarter have choking or dyspnea and also about a quarter have nocturia four to seven times a night.[13]

The daytime fatigue may be subtle or dangerous, such as falling asleep while driving. It is important for the physician to look for subtle symptoms of driving while tired, such as excessive need for coffee. There are often reductions in dexterity, judgment, memory, and concentration. Patients sometimes report irritability, anxiety, aggressiveness, depression, decreased libido, and erectile dysfunction.

Treatment

The goals of treatment are to establish normal nocturnal oxygenation and ventilation, abolish snoring, and eliminate disruption of sleep due to upper airway closure. Any decision to treat should be based on daytime symptoms and cardiopulmonary function, rather than the RDI. Patients need to avoid factors that increase the severity of upper airway obstruction (e.g., sleep deprivation, heavy alcohol use especially near bedtime, sedatives, and obesity).

Continuous Positive Airway Pressure

Most patients will also need nasally applied continuous positive airway pressure (CPAP). This is the "gold standard" of treatment of OSAS. It provides a pneumatic splint for the collapsed pharyngeal airway of sleep apnea. CPAP quickly corrects the anatomy of the airway, improves sleep efficiency, and reduces the cardiovascular risk and daytime somnolence found in this syndrome.

Oral Appliances

Oral appliances can effectively treat snoring and mild to moderate OSAS. There are many appliances that can change the three-dimensional configuration of the airway. Patients often prefer them instead of CPAP, but they are not uniformly effective.

Surgical Therapy

Surgical therapy is invasive and not uniformly effective. There are several surgical options. Nasal reconstruction is the most commonly used. Very rarely, even tracheostomy is needed for patients with morbid obesity with severe hypoxemia. Tonsillectomy is typically curative for children with sleep apnea from adenotonsillar hypertrophy.

Restless Legs Syndrome

Patients with restless legs syndrome (RLS) have dysesthetic sensations at rest. These sensations are described as "pins and needles" or as "creepy, crawly" sensations. There is an almost irresistible urge to move the legs trying to find relief. Symptoms are usually worse later in the day and at bedtime. They sometimes awaken the patient from sleep. The sleep disruption that sometimes occurs can cause daytime somnolence.

RLS is a common disorder. Epidemiologic studies have indicated that 2% to 15% of the population may experience RLS symptoms.[14] Primary RLS is a central nervous system disorder with a high familial incidence. Secondary causes of RLS are also important. Iron deficiency, even without anemia, as demonstrated by a low serum ferritin level (<50 μg/L) can cause RLS. Up to 19% of women during pregnancy develop RLS. It usually subsides within a few weeks postpartum. Spinal cord and peripheral nerve lesions as well as uremia and certain medications, including tricyclic antidepressants, as well as selective serotonin reuptake antagonists, lithium, and dopamine antagonists can also cause RLS.

Diagnosis

A sleep study is not usually indicated in the workup of RLS. Laboratory tests include serum ferritin and serum chemistry tests to rule out uremia, diabetes, and hypothyroidism.

Treatment

Nonpharmacologic treatment includes reduction in caffeine and alcohol intake and cessation of smoking. Drug treatment of RLS can be challenging. L-dopa with carbidopa (Sinemet one-half to one 25/100 mg tablet before bedtime can be helpful. Sometimes a middle of the night dose is needed. Dopamine agonists such as pergolide (Permax) and pramipexole (Mirapex) are also useful. Mirapex is better tolerated and used in doses of 0.375 to 1.5 mg per night. This class of drugs is highly effective, but the role of their long-term use is unknown.[15] They can cause severe nausea and more importantly, sleepiness, which has been reported to be severe enough to cause automobile accidents.[16] They need careful dosing to optimize symptom control and minimize side effects. Opioids including codeine, hydrocodone, oxycodone, propoxyphene, and tramadol can be used intermittently or continuously. Tolerance and dependance can occur. Benzodiazepines such as clonazepam and temazepam are helpful when other medications are not tolerated. Anticonvulsants such as carbamazepine and gabapentin are considered when dopamine agonists have failed. They are most helpful with coexisting peripheral neuropathy.[17]

Augmentation is a worsening of RLS symptoms in the course of therapy. Typically, symptoms can occur earlier in the day than before therapy began. It can occur at any time in the course of RLS therapy. Augmentation has been reported with dopamine agonists and may occur with other medications.[17]

Periodic Movements During Sleep

Almost all patients with RLS also have stereotyped repetitive movements during sleep. These are called periodic leg movements during sleep (PLMS). These movements consist of extensions of the big toe and dorsiflexions of the ankle with occasional flexions of the knee and hip. They last about 0.5 to 5.0 seconds, recur about every 20 seconds, and cluster into episodes lasting minutes or hours.

References

1. Cauter EV, Leproult R, Plat L. Age-related changes in slow wave sleep and REM sleep and relationship with growth hormone and cortisol levels in healthy men. JAMA 2000;284:861–8.
2. National Heart, Lung and Blood Institute Working Group on Insomnia. Insomnia: assessment and management in primary care. Am Fam Physician 1999;59:3029–38.
3. Edinger JD, Wohlegemuth WK, Radtke RA, Marsh GR, Quillian RE. Cognitive behavioral therapy for treatment of chronic primary insomnia. JAMA 2001;285:1856–64.
4. Walsh JK, Roth T, Randazzo A, et al. Eight weeks of non-nightly use of zolpidem for primary insomnia. Sleep 2000;23:1087–96.
5. Roth T. New trends in insomnia management. J Psychopharmacol 1999;13:S37–40.
6. Medical Letter consultants. Hypnotic Drugs. Med Lett Drugs Ther 2000;42:71–2.
7. Ancoli-Israel S. Insomnia in the elderly: a review for the primary care practitioner. Sleep 2000;23:S23–30.
8. Sack RI, Brandes RW, Kendall AR, Lewy AJ. Entrainment of free-running circadian rhythms by melatonin in blind people. N Engl J Med 2000;343:1070–7.
9. Medical Letter consultants. Modafinil for narcolepsy. Med Lett Drugs Ther 1999;41:30–1.
10. Young T, Palta M, Dempsey J, et al. The occurrence of sleep-disordered breathing among middle-aged adults. N Engl J Med 1993;328:1230–5.
11. He J, Meier H, Kryger MR, et al. Mortality and apnea index in obstructive sleep apnea; experience in 385 male patients. Chest 1988;94:9–14.
12. Fletcher EC. The relationship between systemic hypertension and obstructive sleep apnea: facts and theory. Am J Med 1995;98:118–28.

13. Hoffstein V, Szalai JP. Predictive value of clinical features in diagnosing obstructive sleep apnea. Sleep 1993;16:118–22.
14. Lavigne GJ, Montplaisir JY. Restless legs syndrome and sleep bruxism: prevalence and association among Canadians. Sleep 1994;17(8):739–43.
15. Montplaisir J, Nicolas A, Denesle R, et al. Restless legs syndrome improved by pramipexole. A double blind randomized trial. Neurology 1999;52:938–43.
16. Frucht S, Rogers JD, Greene PE, et al. Falling asleep at the wheel: motor vehicle mishaps in persons taking pramipexole and ropinirole. Neurology 1999;52:1908–10.
17. National Center on Sleep Disorder Research, NHLBI, NIH. Restless legs syndrome. Detection and management in primary care. NIH publication no. 00-3788, March 2000.

7
Care of the Alcoholic Patient

Gerald M. Cross, Kenneth A. Hirsch, and John P. Allen

The abuse of alcohol is one of the major health problems in our society. Individuals with alcohol problems are disproportionately represented in the primary care population. In that setting, 11% to 20% of patients meet diagnostic criteria for alcohol dependence or abuse.[1] The family physician's role in the care of patients with alcohol problems may include screening, brief intervention, identification of affected family members, pharmacotherapy, detoxification, treatment of associated medical problems, and referral for consultation and rehabilitation.[2]

Background

Prevalence

Misuse of alcohol has a dramatic impact on many facets of life. The economic burden to society of alcohol abuse exceeds that of either illicit drugs or tobacco. The annual cost to U.S. society associated with alcohol abuse has been estimated as $184.6 billion for 1998. The major economic impact of alcohol abuse is on productivity losses due to alcohol-related illness and premature death. Over $26 billion of the total cost of alcohol abuse derives from treatment and prevention.[3] Annually, more than 100,000 deaths are believed to be alcohol-related.

Table 7.1. **Definitions**

Adult children of alcoholics (ACOA): This group has an increased risk for alcohol problems and may have personality traits such as perfectionistic attitude with low self-esteem.

Alcohol: Refers to ethanol.

Alcohol abuse: *Diagnostic and Statistical Manual of Mental Disorders* (DSM) category for individuals who suffer adverse consequences of drinking that are not sufficient to meet the definition for alcohol dependence.

Alcohol dependence: A group of cognitive, behavioral, and physiologic symptoms defined by the DSM. It encompasses individuals who are unable to control their drinking despite the adverse consequences of drinking.

Alcoholic: Used as the equivalent of the DSM diagnosis of alcohol dependence.

Binge drinking: Five or more drinks at a single setting.

Blackout: Anterograde amnesia associated with drinking.

Co-dependent: Usually a nonalcoholic family member who suffers as a result of the alcoholic's behavior and who attempts to control that behavior.

Cross-tolerance: Tolerance often carries over to other drugs of the same class.

Enabler: A spouse, friend, coworker, physician, or other individual who makes excuses for the alcoholic's behavior so the alcoholic does not have to face the consequences of his or her drinking.

Heavy drinking: Fourteen or more drinks per week.

Kindling: Phenomenon of progressively increased neuroexcitation during repeated withdrawals.

One drink: Equivalent to 12 ounces regular beer, 5–6 ounces wine, or 1.5 ounces "hard liquor."

Tolerance: The individual requires larger amounts of alcohol to produce the same effect. It is partially due to accelerated liver metabolism of alcohol and cellular resistance to alcohol's effects.

Approximately 7.4% of Americans meet the diagnostic criteria for alcohol abuse or alcoholism (Table 7.1).[2] Their medical care costs up to three times more than that of the general population.[4] Fifty percent of all alcohol is consumed by 10% of the drinking population. More people drink heavily in the 21- to 34-year age group, and the fewest people drink heavily in the over 65 age group.[5]

Specific Populations

Ethnicity

Employment status, ethnicity, age, and gender influence the severity of alcohol abuse and treatment outcome. African-American men have only a slightly higher incidence of drug and alcohol disorders than do Caucasian men.[6] Among these two groups employment status was a better predictor of the severity of alcohol problems than was race.[7] American-Hispanic teenagers drink more heavily than either their African-American or Caucasian age peers, and Hispanic men suffer more alcohol-related problems than either African-American or Caucasian men. Alcohol abuse is a particularly serious problem for Native Americans. Although drinking behavior varies widely from tribe to tribe, most Native-American families are affected by alcoholism. Accidents, liver disease, homicide, and suicide, all of which may be alcohol related, rank among the top 10 causes of Native-American mortality.[6] Asian Americans have the lowest level of alcohol consumption and the lowest frequency of alcohol-related problems of any ethnic group in the United States. Within this group, drinking seems to be more socially controlled. Genetic factors may also diminish the risk of alcohol problems in this group.

Age

Overall, the earlier the age when drinking begins, the greater the long-term risk of alcohol abuse. Those who begin drinking during pre- and early adolescence are more likely to develop an alcohol disorder.[8] Many children and adolescents fall into this group. Among high school seniors, 80% report that they have already used alcohol, and 33% report having been drunk in the past 30 days.[3] Compared to parental influence, peer group norms more strongly influence the adolescent's drinking behavior. An adolescent's involvement with alcohol and tobacco serves as a predictor of subsequent experimentation with other illicit drugs.[9] Alcohol-associated violence and vehicular accidents have become the leading cause of death for America's youth.[9] Suicide victims often have a positive blood alcohol concentration (BAC). Unlike older patients, adolescents usually present psychosocial rather than physical signs of alcohol abuse. Elderly people typically drink less alcohol than do young people. Reduced consumption among older individuals may be due to health problems, decreased income, or changes in metabolism and the distribution of alcohol (higher BAC for equivalent amount of alcohol consumed). The combined use of medications and alcohol is a particular risk for elderly patients. Alcohol interacts with medications and can alter the effects of medication, especially in this age group (Table 7.2).

Gender

Men and women have differences in the way they absorb and metabolize alcohol. After consuming the same amount of alcohol,

Table 7.2. **Selected Alcohol–Drug and Alcohol–Herbal Interactions**

Anesthetics	
Propofol (Diprivan)	Increased dose required to produce unconsciousness in chronic drinkers
Enflurane (Ethrane)	Greater risk of liver damage in chronic drinkers
Halothane (Fluothane)	Greater risk of liver damage in chronic drinkers
Antibiotics	
Furazolidone (Furoxone)	Increased risk of nausea, vomiting, headache, and convulsions with acute alcohol consumption
Griseofulvin (Grisactin)	Increased risk of nausea, vomiting, headache, and convulsions with acute alcohol consumption
Metronidazole (Flagyl)	Disulfiram-like reaction; increased risk of nausea, vomiting, headache, and convulsions with acute alcohol consumption
Isoniazid	Decreased availability in the bloodstream with acute alcohol consumption
Rifampin	Decreased availability in the bloodstream with chronic alcohol consumption
Anticoagulants	
Warfarin (Coumadin)	Increased risk of hemorrhages due to increased warfarin availability with acute alcohol consumption; chronic alcohol consumption decreases warfarin availability
Antidepressants	
Amitriptyline (Elavil)	Alcohol increases sedative effect
Monoamine oxidase (MAO) inhibitors	Tyramine found in some beers and wine may produce a dangerous rise in blood pressure
Antidiabetic	
Tolbutamide (Orinase)	Increased availability with acute alcohol consumption and decreased availability with chronic consumption
Antihistamines	
Diphenhydramine (Benadryl)	Increased sedation with acute alcohol consumption

(continued)

Table 7.2 (Continued).

Antipsychotic	
Chlorpromazine (Thorazine)	Increased sedation with acute alcohol consumption; possible liver damage with chronic alcohol consumption
Antiseizure	
Phenytoin (Dilantin)	Increased availability with acute alcohol consumption; chronic drinking decreases availability
Cardiovascular	
Nitroglycerin	Vasodilation; acute alcohol consumption may cause fainting upon standing up
Propranolol (Inderal)	Chronic alcohol consumption decreases availability
Disulfiram	Aldehyde dehydrogenase inhibition produces nausea, vomiting, and potentially shock in the presence of alcohol
Humulus lupulus (Hops)	May potentiate other sedative medications
Narcotics	Increased sedative effect with alcohol
Nonnarcotic pain relievers	
Aspirin	Increased risk of gastric bleeding with alcohol; aspirin may heighten the effects of alcohol
Acetaminophen (Tylenol)	Chronic alcohol consumption increases the risk of liver damage
Oenotherabiennis (evening primrose oil)	Caution if used in patients taking drugs that may lower seizure threshold
Piper methysticum (Kava-Kava)	May potentiate benzodiazepines, alcohol and other central nervous system depressants.
Sedative/hypnotics	
Benzodiazepines	Increased sedation with alcohol; increased risk of accidents, especially in older patients
Barbiturates	Acute alcohol consumption prolongs sedative effects; chronic alcohol use decreases availability of barbiturates due to enzyme activation
Valerian officinalis (Valerian)	May potentiate sedatives and barbiturates

women reach a higher blood alcohol concentration, probably due to their smaller amount of body water and due to a lower activity of the enzyme alcohol dehydrogenase (ADH). These differences make women more susceptible to alcohol-induced liver and heart damage.[10] Women also experience a modest dose-response relationship between breast cancer and alcohol consumption.[3] Alcohol metabolism alters the balance of reproductive hormones, decreasing testosterone levels in men and increasing estradiol levels in women.

Throughout all age groups, men are two to five times more likely to be "problem drinkers" than are women. Although women drink less alcohol than men, they and their children are often the victims of family members who abuse alcohol.[6] Women who enter the labor force tend to drink somewhat more alcohol than other women.[11]

Etiology

Several models have been proposed to explain alcoholism.[12] Historically, the moral model has influenced Western culture. This model views alcoholism as a character weakness and recommends willpower as the solution for alcohol problems. Some proponents of this model remain, and the United States Supreme Court once labeled alcoholism "willful misconduct." The learning model provides another view of alcoholism, describing it as a maladaptive habit. The model contends that new learning can reverse the habit. Although this model is generally consistent with a goal of complete abstinence, it raises the unfortunate belief that the alcohol-dependent patient can someday resume drinking safely.

Today a modified or developmental disease model provides a widely accepted explanation of alcoholism.[13] Alcoholism is viewed as a complex disorder influenced by environmental and genetic influences. The goal of treatment is complete abstinence. Although not without criticism, the disease model has the advantage that it avoids blame and supports treatment. As with other diseases, biopsychosocial factors (ethnicity, age, gender, environment, genetics) and personal choices can affect the onset and outcome of alcoholism. Related to this is the concept of problematic alcohol use developing as a consequence of depression, e.g., self-medication. To the extent that this is valid for a given patient, treatment for depression as an independent disease entity becomes crucial.

Evidence that a significant portion of our vulnerability to alcoholism is genetic has greatly influenced the direction of alcohol research and established a biologic basis of alcoholism.[3] Twin and adoption studies suggest a genetic predisposition to alcoholism and pattern of alcohol consumption. A study of Finnish twins[14] revealed that the quantity of alcohol consumed over a period of 6 years was influenced more by heredity than by environmental factors. The genetic predisposition to alcohol abuse may also be related to alcohol sensitivity due to genetic variants in metabolism of acetaldehyde, as is found in the Chinese Han people. A variant form of the enzyme aldehyde dehydrogenase-2 (ALDH2) has a dominant inheritance pattern and results in slower clearing of acetaldehyde.[13] This sensitivity to alcohol results in rapid flushing, which may protect against heavy or frequent use.[15] Attention has focused on serotonin (5-hydroxytryptamine, 5-HT) dysfunction as part of the biologic basis of alcoholism. 5-HT modulates impulse control and mood. Substantial evidence points to defects in 5-HT neurotransmission in alcoholics, generally indicating that alcoholics have decreased 5-HT neurotransmission.[16] Predisposition toward alcoholism is clearly not predestination for alcoholism, but a family history of alcoholism does increase the vulnerability to developing it. As with atherosclerosis and other diseases, individuals with a positive family history for alcoholism can modify their behavior to decrease their risk of alcohol dependence. Early tolerance may be a marker for a genetically related increased risk of alcoholism.[17]

Physiology

Alcohol is absorbed through the gastrointestinal tract, largely metabolized in the liver, and goes on to affect every organ system. Alcohol absorption is increased when concentrated drinks are taken on an empty stomach. Food (especially fat) in the stomach slows alcohol absorption by dilution and by delayed emptying into the small intestine where absorption is faster. Alcohol passes through the liver before it reaches the circulatory system. High concentrations of alcohol exceed the metabolic capacity of the liver, allowing more alcohol to reach the blood and brain. Typically, after one standard drink (12 ounces of beer, 5 ounces of wine, or 1.5 ounces of 80-proof distilled spirit), the BAC will peak within 30 to 45 minutes.

Alcohol metabolism proceeds at a constant rate (zero-order kinetics). Alcohol is first metabolized to acetaldehyde. The ADH enzyme carries out most of this metabolic step, but there are genetic variations in its activity. With chronic exposure to alcohol, the microsomal ethanol-oxidizing system (MEOS), another metabolic pathway for alcohol, may accelerate the rate of metabolism. Although individuals vary greatly in their ability to metabolize alcohol, an average man can metabolize about 10 mL of absolute alcohol (or one drink) per hour.

Acetaldehyde is subsequently metabolized to acetate owing to the action of aldehyde dehydrogenase. Disulfiram (Antabuse) inhibits several enzymes that metabolize acetalde-hyde. In the presence of alcohol, disulfiram causes acetaldehyde to accumulate, leading to flushing, tachycardia, nausea, vomiting, and later a drop in blood pressure. These signs and symptoms are referred to as the disulfiram-ethanol reaction.

About 5% to 10% of alcohol is released unchanged in breath and urine. Alcohol in alveolar air correlates directly with the arterial BAC, whereas levels in urine correlate with the current level of intoxication only if the bladder is emptied and the subsequent urine is tested.

Alcohol interacts with both water and lipids, allowing it to penetrate and disorder cell membranes. There is no blood–brain barrier to alcohol. Because of the brain's vascularity, the concentration of alcohol in the brain may in fact exceed the level in the venous peripheral blood until the alcohol equilibrates in total body water. Until this balance is reached, the blood alcohol concentration may be less than the cerebrospinal fluid (CSF) concentration.[18] The placenta is unable to protect the fetus from exposure to alcohol in the mother's blood. Similarly, breast milk conveys some of the alcohol in the mother's blood to the infant.

Clinical Presentation

Mental Status

In the emergency room, intoxicated patients often present with a history of recent drinking and demonstrate socially inappropriate behavior, impaired judgment, and altered consciousness. Hospitalized patients who show mental status impairment combined with sympathetic signs should be evaluated for withdrawal from alcohol, other sedative-hypnotics, or both. These patients may have anterograde amnesia, referred to as a blackout. Head trauma should be ruled out by both examination and by the patient's own report. Serial mental status examinations using a standardized format such as the Mini-Mental Status Examination are needed until substantial cognitive clearing is demonstrated. Alcoholics may present with frank delirium (altered consciousness, impaired attention, sleep–wake cycle disturbance, cognitive disorganization, dysperceptions), dementia (intellectual decline and personality changes resulting in social impairment), or both. Fluctuation in the patient's level of functioning argues for delirium, which should be considered a medical emergency until the etiology is clearly identified. To differentiate between delirium and a psychotic disorder, a generally valid guideline is that the predominance of visual or tactile hallucinations suggests an organic etiology (e.g., delirium), whereas predominantly auditory hallucinations are more suggestive of a psychotic disorder.

Many alcoholics appear anxious or depressed, conditions that often resolve after detoxification. Sometimes clinical depression coexists with or underlies alcoholism. If depression does not diminish within several weeks of drinking cessation, treatment with an antidepressant is recommended. Treatment of primary depression may reduce the risk of a return to drinking because of continued depression, and if treatment is with a serotonergic agent, craving for alcohol (and other drugs) may be reduced, further promoting abstinence.

Brain

Chronic alcoholics lose both gray and white matter volumes. Neuronal damage may result from increased levels of reactive oxygen species and lipid peroxidation products, exceeding the capacity of the body's normal nucleotide excision repair of damaged DNA.[19] Organic brain syndromes among alcohol-dependent patients can usually be categorized as Wernicke-Korsakoff syndrome or alcoholic dementia. Wernicke's disease includes a triad of signs: confusion, ocular disturbances, and ataxia, caused by thiamine deficiency. Korsakoff's psychosis may be the chronic phase of Wernicke's disease. It includes impaired recent memory and the inability to learn new information. Confabulation, or making up details to fill in gaps in memory, has been associated with Korsakoff's psychosis. Alcoholic dementia includes total intellectual decline with dysphasia, apraxia, and cerebral atrophy. This condition may be difficult to distinguish from Alzheimer's disease. The long-term effect of alcohol on the brain, even after prolonged abstinence, is demonstrated by the extreme rapidity with which tolerance is redeveloped if the patient returns to drinking.

Neurotransmitter function constitutes an important area of alcohol research. Broadly summarized, it appears that withdrawal phenomena are mediated by dopaminergic pathways, pleasure from alcohol and drugs (and other stimuli) by opioid pathways, and craving by serotonergic pathways. This hypothesis has given rise to potential treatment options (discussed under Management, below).

Liver

Alcohol is hepatotoxic even in the presence of adequate nutrition. A single weekend of heavy drinking may be all that is necessary to produce a fatty liver. This may represent a stress reaction, as the adrenals contribute to the mobilization of fatty acids while the liver is occupied metabolizing alcohol. Continued drinking may produce alcoholic hepatitis. Whereas the fatty liver is asymptomatic, alcoholic hepatitis produces jaundice, fever, and loss of appetite. The size of the liver may increase, and enzyme levels may be elevated. Liver biopsy may reveal polymorphonuclear leukocytes and necrosis near the central vein. A typical, but nonspecific, feature of hepatocytes damaged by alcohol is the Mallory body, a hyaline inclusion. These effects on the liver may be due to the combination of a hepatic hypermetabolic state following alcohol exposure and inadequate oxygenation. Necrosis appears where the oxygen tension is lowest. Whereas fatty liver and alcoholic hepatitis are reversible, cirrhosis is not. It develops after continued necrosis and scar formation. The cirrhotic liver tends to be small and hard. Histologic findings of fatty liver, alcoholic hepatitis, and cirrhosis can be found concurrently in the same patient.[20] Although the risk of cirrhosis is a function of the amount of alcohol consumed, individual susceptibility also plays a role, and only about 10% of heavy drinkers develop clinically apparent cirrhosis.

The high prevalence of hepatitis C in the substance abusing population complicates the medical status of patients, their efforts at abstinence, and their psychiatric status (the latter adversely impacted by interferon treatment).

Pancreas

Acute pancreatitis seems to occur randomly among heavily drinking men.[21] The combination of heavy alcohol consumption, increased amylase, upper abdominal pain, nausea, and vomiting suggest the diagnosis, but it can be confirmed only at laparotomy or autopsy. The absence of an elevated amylase level does not rule out the diagnosis. Some alcoholics have an increased amylase level in the absence of pancreatitis due to amylase from the salivary glands. Radiographic findings may include a sentinel loop. Acute hemorrhagic pancreatitis can be fatal. Acute pancreatitis may be a separate entity or the early stage of chronic alcoholic pancreatitis. Seventy-five percent of cases of chronic pancreatitis in the United States are related to alcohol abuse.[21] Deep epigastric pain radiating to the back following alcohol ingestion or a heavy meal is the characteristic presentation. There may be few physical findings. Amylase levels may be normal. Ultrasonography, computed tomography, and endoscopic retrograde pancreatography are useful tests for confirming the diagnosis. Relief of pain and abstinence from alcohol are the foundation for the treatment of chronic alcoholic pancreatitis. Abstinence may allow the patient to avoid more severe disease but does not necessarily normalize pancreatic function.

Prenatal Effects

Alcohol consumption during the first trimester is associated with multiple fetal anomalies. Exposure during the second and third trimesters is associated with growth retardation and neurobehavioral changes such as sleep disturbances and decreased attentiveness. Moderate to heavy drinking pregnant women experience a two- to fourfold increase in the incidence of second trimester spontaneous abortions. Fetal alcohol syndrome (FAS) describes a set of fetal abnormalities associated with alcohol consumption during pregnancy. The prevalence of FAS in the United States ranges from 0.5 to 3.0 per 1000 live births, and higher in some populations.[3] Criteria for FAS are prenatal or postnatal growth retardation (or both), central nervous system (CNS) involvement, and specific craniofacial dysmorphic features (microcephaly, hypoplastic maxilla, thinned upper lip, short upturned nose, and short palpebral fissure). Facial features associated with FAS tend to disappear during adulthood. Until recently, infants of alcoholic mothers who partially meet the criteria were diagnosed as having fetal alcohol effect (FAE). The Institute of Medicine of the National Academy of Sciences has classified prenatal alcohol exposure into five categories. Three categories represent children who have all or some of the FAS facial features. The other two categories do not have FAS facial features: alcohol-related neurodevelopmental disorder (ARND) and alcohol-related birth defects (ARBDs). Magnetic resonance imaging (MRI) scans of children with FAS show proportionally reduced basal ganglia, a smaller corpus callosum and cerebellum. The peak BAC contributes more to the development of FAS than does the amount consumed.[6] The more severe morphologic defects occur with more extreme levels of alcohol consumption. There is substantial individual variation in susceptibility to alcohol's effect on the fetus. Not all women who drink heavily deliver FAS infants, but no ethnic or racial group is invulnerable to the teratogenic effect of alcohol.[22] In light of the severity of the risk of FAS, it is not yet possible to recommend that any level of alcohol consumption is safe for a pregnant woman.

Cardiac Effects: Risk Versus Benefit

Advice to patients should include a discussion of the potential risks and benefits associated with alcohol consumption. Caucasian-

American men who report drinking fewer than three drinks per day were found to be less likely to die over a 12-year follow-up period than men who reported complete abstinence. Meta-analysis found that the lowest overall mortality for men was associated with an alcohol consumption of 10 g (less than one drink) per day for men and less for women. At 20 g of alcohol per day (between one and two drinks) women had an overall mortality significantly higher than abstainers.[3] The improved outcome is primarily associated with reduced coronary artery disease. Some risks of alcohol consumption may occur at moderate levels of consumption, including hemorrhagic stroke, vehicular accidents, harmful interactions with more than 100 medications and alternative medications, a 50% increase in breast cancer among women drinking three to nine drinks per week, and decreased intelligence quotient (IQ) of children born to mothers reporting as few as two drinks per day while pregnant. Heavy alcohol consumption over a period of years is associated with heart failure secondary to cardiomyopathy and susceptibility to a variety of other illnesses including tuberculosis (TB) and human immunodeficiency virus (HIV). Binge drinking has been associated with cardiac dysrhythmias, especially atrial fibrillation.

Physicians should inform their patients about these known trade-offs. Individuals who have a very low risk of heart disease are unlikely to experience reduced mortality from moderate drinking. The reverse appears to be true for those with a high risk of heart disease. Individuals with a family history of alcoholism should be frankly discouraged from drinking. The National Institute of Alcohol Abuse and Alcoholism recommends that people 65 and older limit their alcohol consumption to one drink per day.

Diagnosis

Alcoholics may be difficult to identify, and collateral information is often critical for evaluating the patient's history. Alcoholics often minimize alcohol's impact on their life, but collateral information from family and friends typically reveals personal and marital problems related to drinking. During any routine medical examination all adolescents and adults should be asked about alcohol use. No single symptom or test can diagnose alcoholism, although the screening tests described below[23,24] are useful. Screening may itself be beneficial by drawing the patient's attention to problems related to drinking, and it may promote self-monitoring and behavioral change.[25] The diagnostic criteria in the *Diagnostic and Statistical Manual of Mental Disorders*, 4th edition (DSM-IV)[26] (Table 7.3). defines alcohol abuse

Table 7.3. **Diagnosis of Alcohol Use Disorders**

Alcohol abuse

For a diagnosis of alcohol abuse the patient must show one or more of the following, related to alcohol, on a recurrent basis:
1. Failure to fulfill major role obligations
2. Use in physically hazardous situations
3. Legal problems
4. Continued use despite having persistent or recurrent social or interpersonal problems related to alcohol use

Alcohol dependence

For a diagnosis of alcohol dependence at least three of these seven criteria must be met:
1. Clinically significant tolerance[a]
2. Clinically significant withdrawal
3. Recurrent failure of intent
4. Recurrent failure of control
5. Preoccupation with alcohol
6. Predominance of alcohol-related activities
7. Continued alcohol use despite knowledge that the drinking contributes to a psychological, physical, social, or other problem

[a]It is noteworthy that tolerance to some effects of alcohol (e.g., gait, coordination) does not necessarily suggest tolerance to all effects. Certain effects, especially impaired social judgment, may demonstrate little or no tolerance.

Source: American Psychiatric Association,[5] with permission.

as recurrent problems in one or more of the four areas of functioning; dependence is defined by the presence of at least three of seven specific areas of dysfunction.

Screening

A variety of self-report instruments are available to screen for alcohol problems.[27] Administration times generally range from less than a minute to about 5 minutes. Perhaps the most common measure is the CAGE, an acronym for the key word in each of four questions related to drinking[28]:

1. Have you ever felt you should *C*ut down on your drinking?
2. Have people *A*nnoyed you by criticizing your drinking?
3. Have you ever felt *G*uilty about your drinking?
4. Have you ever had a drink first thing in the morning to steady your nerves or to get rid of a hangover (*E*ye-opener)?

Despite its popularity and brevity, the CAGE has certain limitations. In particular, it focuses on emotional reactions to drinking and asks about lifetime occurrence of symptoms rather than recent events.

The Michigan Alcoholism Screening Test (MAST)[29] and variants are also commonly used in primary care settings. This family of instruments has been criticized for focusing too heavily on late-stage symptoms such as liver pathology and delirium tremens. Furthermore, as with the CAGE, the questions on the MAST do not specify when the symptoms occurred, thus causing individuals with earlier, resolved problems to still score positively. Nevertheless, the CAGE, the MAST, and similar scales have fairly high validity.

A newer measure, the Alcohol Use Disorders Identification Test (AUDIT)[30] merits particular attention from primary care physicians (Table 7.4). Its advantages are brevity (approximately 2 minutes), focus on the preceding year, and item sampling from several domains

Table 7.4. **Alcohol Use Disorders Identification Test (AUDIT) Questionnaire**

1. How often do you have a drink containing alcohol?
   (0) Never
   (1) Monthly or less
   (2) Two to four times a month
   (3) Two or three times a week
   (4) Four or more times a week
2. How many drinks containing alcohol do you have on a typical day when you are drinking?
   (0) 1 or 2
   (1) 3 or 4
   (2) 5 or 6
   (3) 7 or 9
   (4) 10 or more
3. How often do you have six or more drinks on one occasion?
   (0) Never
   (1) Less than monthly
   (2) Monthly
   (3) Weekly
   (4) Daily or almost daily
4. How often during the last year have you found that you were not able to stop drinking once you had started?
   (0) Never
   (1) Less than monthly
   (2) Monthly
   (3) Weekly
   (4) Daily or almost daily

(*continued*)

Table 7.4 (Continued).

---

5. How often during the last year have you failed to do what was normally expected from you because of drinking?
   (0) Never
   (1) Less than monthly
   (2) Monthly
   (3) Weekly
   (4) Daily or almost daily
6. How often during the last year have you needed a first drink in the morning to get yourself going after a heavy drinking session?
   (0) Never
   (1) Less than monthly
   (2) Monthly
   (3) Weekly
   (4) Daily or almost daily
7. How often during the last year have you had a feeling of guilt or remorse after drinking?
   (0) Never
   (1) Less than monthly
   (2) Monthly
   (3) Weekly
   (4) Daily or almost daily
8. How often during the last year have you been unable to remember what happened the night before because you had been drinking?
   (0) Never
   (1) Less than monthly
   (2) Monthly
   (3) Weekly
   (4) Daily or almost daily
9. Have you or someone else been injured as a result of your drinking?
   (0) No
   (2) Yes, but not in the last year
   (4) Yes, during the last year
10. Has a relative, friend, doctor, or other health worker been concerned about your drinking or suggested that you should cut down?
    (0) No
    (2) Yes, but not in the last year
    (4) Yes, during the last year

Numbers in parentheses are scoring weights. The usual cutoff for the AUDIT to be scored as positive is 8 points.

(intake, level of dependence, and adverse consequences of drinking). The AUDIT can be embedded in a general health risk appraisal survey dealing with other medical concerns such as smoking, diet, and nutrition. In a recent review contrasting it with other self-report alcohol screening measures, the AUDIT tended to perform best. A cutoff score of 6 points for females may be preferable to the more common research cutoff of 8.[31]

History

The history should include what the patient drinks, how much, how often, when alcohol was last drunk, and if the patient has used any other drugs or medications. Patients in denial minimize their drinking history. It is therefore important to review the history with the patient's family members or friends. The focus should not be on whether the individual has a problem with alcohol, but rather on the consequences of drinking (e.g., legal, financial, medical, social difficulties). Asking if others believe the patient has a problem or that drinking contributes to a social problem may be more effective than direct questions about the patient's drinking. It is important to inquire about previous withdrawal history, as successive withdrawals tend to become more severe.

Laboratory Tests

Laboratory tests can be used for screening and to support the diagnosis. Such tests might include measuring the BAC, a urine drug screen, bilirubin assay, prothrombin time, assays of liver-associated enzymes, electrolytes, and a complete blood count. Elevation of the bilirubin, liver-associated enzymes, and prothrombin time suggests the presence of liver dysfunction. Increased mean corpuscular volume (MCV) and mean corpuscular hemoglobin (MCH) and a decreased red blood cell (RBC) count suggest that the patient has been drinking heavily for weeks or months. MCV changes may persist for months.

The half-life of γ-glutamyltransferase (GGT) is approximately 26 days, and an elevated GGT level may be one of the most sensitive laboratory screening tests for alcoholism. An elevated carbohydrate-deficient transferrin (CDT) level is the most sensitive indicator of relapse to drinking in a purportedly abstinent patient.[23] Unlike the other biochemical markers, a rise in CDT does not seem to reflect organ damage, but rather recent heavy (five drinks or more per day) consumption of alcohol. (CDT was recently approved by the Food and

Drug Administration as an indicator of excessive drinking, the first alcohol biomarker so approved.) An elevated aspartate transferase/ alanine transferase (AST/ALT) ratio (e.g., 2:1 or higher) has been interpreted as evidence of liver disease secondary to drinking alcohol, whereas a reversed ratio (e.g. 1:2) has been seen as evidence of hepatitis due to other causes. This "rule" may not hold true for all populations. The simultaneous use of CDT and GGT assays to screen for excessive alcohol consumption seems reasonably sensitive (75%) and specific (85%). Ultimately, the diagnosis of alcohol dependence must meet the criteria established by the DSM-IV.[26]

Management

Intervention

The physician should give clear directions to the patient to reduce alcohol consumption, usually in the context of health, social, or family problems.[2] The goal is to present information about the illness in a manner that can be understood and accepted by the alcoholic. A more formal intervention may include gathering friends, family members, and even the employer to firmly confront the alcoholic's behavior. The goal of this type of intervention is to obtain the alcoholic's agreement to enter treatment that same day. To be successful, this procedure often requires hours of preparation before the intervention takes place. Some treatment programs assist the physician and family in preparing the intervention. The intervention is a powerful tool that often succeeds in getting the alcoholic patient into treatment. Patients entering treatment as a result of intervention often do as well as those who enter voluntarily.

Comprehensive Assessment

The American Society of Addiction Medicine (ASAM) has released the second version of the patient placement criteria (PPC-II), a tool to help the clinician utilize the data from a comprehensive assessment to determine the appropriate level of care for a particular patient. Although alcoholism is a primary illness, it is often accompanied by a variety of medical problems (Table 7.5).

Supportive Therapy During Withdrawal

Alcohol withdrawal produces adrenergic arousal. To compensate, the patient's room should be quiet and evenly lit to allow constant re-

Table 7.5. **Summary of Alcohol Effects**

Organ	Acute effect (up to months)	Chronic effects (years)
Breast	Portion of blood alcohol content in breast milk	?Increased risk of breast cancer Male breast enlargement
Cardiovascular system	Moderate blood pressure increase "Holiday heart" syndrome[a]	Hypertension
Central nervous system (CNS)	Impaired motor coordination Sleep apnea	Depression Dementia Peripheral neuropathy Widening of frontal cortical sulci Distal symmetric polyneuropathy Hemorrhagic stroke
Endocrine system	Increased plasma corticosteroids Increased plasma catecholamines	Low testosterone Testicular atrophy Amenorrhea, anovulation
Fetal development	Fetal alcohol syndrome	
Gastrointestinal system	Delayed gastric emptying Gastroesophageal reflux Injures the gastric mucosa Loss of enzymes (disaccharidases) Worsen preexisting peptic ulcers	Esophageal carcinoma Chronic atrophic gastritis ?Gastric carcinoma[b] Esophageal inflammation
Hematopoietic system		Megaloblastic anemia Decreased platelet function

(continued)

Table 7.5 (Continued).

Organ	Acute effect (up to months)	Chronic effects (years)
Immune system		Increased risk of infections
		Decreased production of polymorphonuclear leukocytes
		Decreased cell-mediated immunity
		Decreased T lymphocytes
		Impaired phagocytosis
Liver	Fat deposition	Cirrhosis
	Liver enlargement	Hepatocellular carcinoma[c]
	Alcoholic hepatitis	
Muscular system	Increased chance of muscle injury	Chronic alcoholic myopathy
	Sudden muscle necrosis	
Nutritional system	Interferes with vitamin metabolism	Folate deficiency
	Inhibits gluconeogenesis	Thiamine deficiency
	Indirect loss of calcium and potassium	Alcoholic ketoacidosis
	Loss of magnesium, zinc, and phosphorus	Decreased serum calcium
	Thiamine deficiency	Wernicke-Korsakoff syndrome
Other malignancies		Squamous cell carcinoma of the head and neck
Pancreas	Acute pancreatitis	Chronic pancreatitis
		Pseudocyst formation
Pulmonary system	Increased cough and sputum production	Pneumonia

[a]Holiday heart syndrome refers to atrial or ventricular dysrhythmias following days of heavy drinking.

[b]Smoking may also contribute to the development of gastrointestinal carcinoma.

[c]May be secondary to hepatitis B virus.

orientation to surroundings. Dimming the room lights at night mimics diurnal variation and supports orientation. Staff members should present a pleasant, nonthreatening attitude. Restraints are rarely necessary with proper sedation. Patients may be allowed to eat and drink when they feel ready. Intravenous fluids are usually not necessary for uncomplicated alcohol withdrawal. The medical staff can promote long-term recovery by directing the patient to a rehabilitation program immediately following detoxification. Indeed, some aspects of rehabilitation can be started on the detoxification unit by providing books and tapes, an introduction to an Alcoholics Anonymous (AA) sponsor, and attendance at an AA meeting as soon as the patient is physically able.

Detoxification

Monitored detoxification safely transports the patient through withdrawal. Rehabilitation is the goal; detoxification is a step toward that goal. Detoxification may be done on an inpatient or outpatient basis depending on the clinical presentation and history of the patient. In the context of managed care pressures, outpatient or ambulatory detoxification is becoming more commonplace and appears to work well for many patients.[32] Once detoxified, an alcoholic may still not function well cognitively for days, weeks, or months.

Withdrawal Syndrome

Alcohol withdrawal consists of signs and symptoms ranging from hangover to delirium tremens. The severity depends on the patient's age, physical condition, prior withdrawals, and amount of alcohol consumed. Withdrawal begins as the blood alcohol level falls and includes anxiety, restlessness, insomnia, and nausea. About 24 hours after the last drink (sometimes days longer) the patient may have increased blood pressure and pulse, a low-grade fever, and tremors that increase with the withdrawal severity. Hand tremors may be the most reliable early sign of alcohol withdrawal unless the tremors are reduced by beta-blockers or other medication. Patients in withdrawal may also have tachycardia and dry mouth, which may be misinterpreted as volume depletion. During withdrawal, total body water is more likely to be normal, and plasma volume is likely to be increased.[33] Transient hallucinations may occur that involve any sense, but visual hallucinations are more common. Typically, 2 days after the last drink (but occasionally up to 10 days after the last drink) one or more grand mal seizures occur. Seizures occur in about 5% of untreated withdrawal patients; 30% to 40% of patients with seizures proceed to delirium tremens, typically during the third to fifth day of withdrawal, if adequate treatment is not provided. Delirium tremens is characterized by severe autonomic hyperactivity (e.g., tachycardia, hypertension, fever, diaphoresis, tremor), electrolyte disturbances, hyperreflexia, confusion, disorientation, and clouding of consciousness. Dysperceptions, especially visual and tactile hallucinations, are common, usually without the insight that accompanies hallucinations of milder withdrawal. Delusions are likewise common. Psychomotor activity may fluctuate widely during the course of the delirium, and the patient frequently demonstrates affective lability. Delirium tremens typically persist for 3 to 5 days. Medical management is directed at patient safety, as pharmacologic intervention has not been demonstrated to shorten the duration of the delirium. The physician should be aware that in a debilitated or elderly patient a delirium of any etiology may persist for weeks beyond resolution of the cause of the delirium. Delirium tremens may be fatal, especially in debilitated or elderly patients.

Adolescents often do not develop the classic signs of physical withdrawal seen in adults. They do exhibit the usual behavioral and emotional aspects of dependence. Elderly patients usually have more severe withdrawal than young patients. The rehabilitation progress of elderly patients may be delayed owing to the slower metabolism of medications used to control their alcohol withdrawal.

Pharmacotherapy

The physician should assess the patient's risk of withdrawal before treatment begins. The Clinical Institute Withdrawal Assessment (CIWA)-Ar scale may be used as an adjunct to assess the patient's risk for severe withdrawal.[34] A decision to allow the patient to go through withdrawal without the benefit of medication should be carried out only with informed consent.

Oral multivitamin supplementation, including thiamine, folic acid, and pyridoxine, should be given when the patient can tolerate oral fluids. If intravenous fluids containing dextrose are needed, 100 mg thiamine should be added to each liter of intravenous fluid administered to the patient. A normal magnesium level does not necessarily mean that magnesium supplementation is unnecessary. Serum magnesium levels do not correlate with CSF magnesium levels. Adequate levels of magnesium help prevent cardiac dysrhythmia and seizures. If the clinical history and examination suggest that the patient is at risk for serious withdrawal or is nutritionally compromised, $MgSO_4$ 2 g IM (deep) up to every 8 hours for 2 to 3 days may be administered.

The pharmacologic basis for detoxification traditionally has been the use of cross-tolerant medication to control alcohol withdrawal. Usually the agent chosen is a benzodiazepine or a barbiturate with a longer biologic half-life than alcohol. Residual symptoms are treated with adjunctive medications (e.g., antiemetic for nausea). Pharmacotherapy is justified to prevent or treat signs and symptoms of withdrawal and possibly to curb alcoholic dementia and kindling.[35] The "kindling" hypothesis suggests that repeated subthreshold (for seizures) stimulation of the CNS during withdrawal increases the risk of subsequent withdrawal seizures. All protocols for the treatment of withdrawal should be modified according to patient needs. Individuals with physical dependence on more than one drug should first be withdrawn from the drug that produces the most dangerous withdrawal. In practice, it may mean withdrawing the patient from sedative-hypnotics (e.g., alcohol) first while medically delaying withdrawal from opiates.

An appropriate benzodiazepine for the treatment of alcohol withdrawal can be selected based on the patient's age and hepatic function. Diazepam is preferred if the patient is under 55 years of age and has a well-functioning liver. Oxazepam is appropriate for older patients and those with liver dysfunction. Diazepam is administered 10 to 20 mg po every hour until the patient's symptoms are relieved and the patient is sedated. Further doses may be unnecessary. Total dosage should not exceed 60 mg without further evaluation by the physician, but doses in excess of 120 mg within 24 hours are not uncommon in the heavy drinker. Patients who are tolerant of alcohol are similarly tolerant of other sedative-hypnotics. Intramuscular chlordiazepoxide is less desirable because of erratic uptake, prolonged metabolism, and delayed onset. Patients requiring high-dose withdrawal pharmacotherapy should be in a monitored bed.

Oxazepam (15–30 mg) may also be given orally every hour until the patient's symptoms are relieved or the patient becomes drowsy. Unlike the diazepam regimen, the cumulative dose of oxazepam necessary to initially relieve the patient's symptoms is repeated every 6 to 8 hours for the remainder of the first day of treatment. The dose is then reduced by 25% on each subsequent day. Most patients complete the regimen by the fifth day.

Phenobarbital remains a reliable, effective medication for the treatment of alcohol withdrawal, for mixed sedative-hypnotic withdrawal, and for seizure prophylaxis when used by experienced clinicians as part of an established protocol. It is easily absorbed. Phenobarbital's effectiveness has been reported to be superior to that of diazepam for delirium tremens.[36] Nervousness or nausea may be treated with promethazine (Phenergan) or hydroxyzine (Atarax, Vistaril). Until recently there was scant literature supporting the use of anticonvulsants in withdrawal treatment, except in the case of an independent seizure disorder. Research supports the clinical efficacy of some agents.[37] For delirious, hallucinating, and combative patients, haloperidol is the agent of choice, in combination with the above withdrawal agents. Haloperidol is safe in oral, intramuscular, and intravenous doses of 70 to 80 mg/day for monitored patients; higher doses are not uncommon. Usually, a dose of just 5 mg orally or intramuscularly two to four times a day is sufficient. The potential of haloperidol to lower seizure threshold is controlled by concomitant administration of an anticonvulsant.

Complications

Seizures are one of the most common complications of alcohol withdrawal. If a seizure occurs, diazepam 5 to 10 mg IV is given until the seizures are controlled or the patient is drowsy but responsive. Causes other than withdrawal should be determined if seizures are associated with head trauma, are not preceded by tremulousness, are focal in nature, or a residual neurologic defect is present.

The combination of liver dysfunction and poor vitamin K absorption can contribute to systemic bleeding. In these circumstances, minor head trauma can lead to a subdural hematoma. This diagnosis should be considered if the patient does not recover as expected.[37] The differential diagnosis for seizures also includes infection and metabolic disturbances.

Keeping the patient in the program during withdrawal is one of the most difficult challenges facing the clinician. Alcoholic patients often have a strong but unrecognized compulsion to leave treatment and return to drinking. Patients who receive adequate medication for withdrawal are less likely to leave "against medical advice." From the first day of treatment, the detoxification unit staff should repeatedly educate the patient that rehabilitation is the treatment goal, not just detoxification. Patients whose urge to leave treatment persists can often be encouraged by concerned family members to persevere.

Rehabilitation

Treatment approaches involving the family tend to be more effective than individual-focused treatment for alcoholics. The family can be used to motivate the patient to enter and stay in treatment. The family can set a common goal, participate in education, and reduce emotional distress. Rehabilitation can be accomplished on an inpatient or outpatient basis or in a partial hospitalization program. Inpatient rehabilitation is preferred for patients who require nursing care or continuous observation, and for those who need an opportunity to progress in an environment that is free of violence and drugs. The severity of alcohol dependence and the absence of an adequate social support system may also justify inpatient treatment. Patients without convenient and reliable transportation may have a better chance of success in an inpatient program. Patients should be individually assessed and given the appropriate level of treatment from the start. The ASAM PPC-II[23] is currently being validated, and it may be used to guide the family physician to select the most appropriate level of treatment for a specific patient. The "first fail" philosophy, which requires patients to fail the least intensive treatment program before they can receive more intensive treatment, may not be cost-effective and is not consistent with quality medical care.

Physical evaluation, psychological assessment, and education of the patient and the patient's family are the foundation of rehabilitation programs. Typically, it is accomplished with group and individual therapy, classes, a family program, and a relapse prevention program. Many programs ascribe to the 12 steps of Alcoholics Anonymous as the philosophic basis of their programs. The long-term success of patients treated in such programs varies,[38] but when there is employer and family support the results can be outstanding.[39]

Continuing Care

An aftercare plan specific to the patient's needs should be created. The family physician should be familiar with this and encourage compliance with the plan. Physicians should generally avoid giving aftercare patients mood-altering medications, as these drugs may increase the chance of relapse. As previously indicated, antidepressants and the opioid antagonists may constitute an exception to this general recommendation. Alcoholism is sometimes associated with a wide range of psychiatric disorders; most notable are mood or affective disorders, anxiety disorders (especially posttraumatic stress disorder), mania, and schizophrenia. When coexisting with another psychiatric disorder, both that disorder and the alcoholism may be exacerbated; both must be treated. Potentially addictive medications should be avoided when treating coexisting psychiatric disorders in alcoholic patients, but rapidly acting benzodiazepines should be specifically avoided. In the event that hospitalization is needed for a condition requiring pain medication or anesthesia, the patient is given medications as necessary, but mood-altering medications are discontinued while the patient is still in the hospital.

Current evidence indicates that serotonin reuptake inhibitors can reduce drinking by heavy drinkers whether or not they are depressed, but the magnitude of the decrease is not dramatic. Placebo-controlled trials showed that naltrexone (ReVia) 50 mg/day could benefit alcoholics in terms of relapse prevention. Naltrexone reduced the number of drinking days and craving for alcohol. Compared to the serotonergic drugs, the opioid antagonists seem to produce more consistent reductions in alcohol consumption.[16] Some aftercare plans include disulfiram in an effort to prevent relapse. If disulfiram is prescribed, specific procedures to ensure compliance are needed. The family physician should educate the patient about food, medications, and cosmetics that contain alcohol and might produce a disulfiram-alcohol reaction. Relapses do occur, and the physician should use such occasions to refocus the continuing care plan for the patient and family.

Prevention

Physicians can play a major role in the prevention and treatment of alcohol-related problems. Training for this role should begin in medical school. Interested faculty members should be offered fellowship training in the study of addiction. Curricula and tests ought to include alcohol-related topics. Medical students and residents should play an integral role on the team that cares for patients in addiction treatment centers. This kind of physician training can support community initiatives for education and social policy changes to prevent alcohol abuse.

Of all the proposed methods to prevent alcohol abuse, education is the least controversial. The most effective educational efforts probably occur during or before adolescence. After that, peer influence becomes more important than parental influence. The physician can support parental norms by teaching adolescents to be comfortable standing up for what they believe. Counseling that delays the onset of drinking until age 15 or later may reduce alcohol related problems.[8] Such "anticipatory guidance" teaches adolescents respect for their own beliefs. The physician can also identify adolescent patients at particularly high risk for alcoholism due to their family backgrounds, peer associations, difficulties in school, or problems with impulse control. These adolescents need specific education concerning the risks of drinking alcohol during pregnancy or while driving.

Social policy changes can support education in preventing alcohol abuse. Several decades ago the price of a beer was a quarter while the price of a soft drink was a nickel. This 5:1 ratio of alcoholic beverage cost to soft drink cost has been lost. The main reason for the change is that taxation on alcoholic beverages has not kept pace with inflation. Today there is near parity in price for these beverages. Social policies that restrict the consumption of alcohol-containing beverages seem to reduce per-capita consumption of alcohol.[40]

Family and Community Issues+

Alcohol-related motor vehicle accidents cause more than 20,000 deaths each year. This toll disproportionately affects young Americans. Nearly half of the violent deaths (accidents, suicide, homicide) among males under age 34 are alcohol-related.[6]

Risks of an automobile accident increase sharply as the BAC rises. Heightened risk begins near 0.04% BAC, and the risk of an accident is doubled at 0.06% BAC. A driver with a BAC of 0.08%, a common legal limit, is six times as likely to have an accident than a sober driver.[18] Raising the drinking age from 18 to 21 years results in decreased alcohol use among high school seniors and an overall decrease in alcohol-related traffic accidents.[41] Raising the legal drinking age has been associated with decreased death rates from automobile accidents, unintentional injuries, and suicide among adolescents and young adults.[42] The single most important deterrent that enhances traffic safety is license suspension.[43] For those convicted of a driving under the influence (DUI) offense, an education program successfully completed may be beneficial; however, the repeat offender also benefits from treatment, including involvement with AA.[44]

Ethical Issues and Physician Responsibilities

Households in which chemicals are abused are at substantially greater risk for both physical and sexual abuse. Neither the victim nor the perpetrator of abuse is likely to speak freely. The victim may experience fear of more severe abuse or even death, abandonment by the abuser, or the shame of being discovered to be a victim. The abuser is fearful of being caught and punished; losing family, job, and freedom; and being publicly humiliated. Honest disclosure by the patient and honest reporting by the physician are also limited by a frequently overlooked factor: in the managed care environment, it is not unusual that payment for services may be denied if the injury has resulted from intoxication. The likelihood of honest disclosure is increased if the physician offers support, hope, and understanding.

There are legal guidelines that govern the physician's actions in the event of threatened suicide or assault, but danger to others may also take the form of an intoxicated patient planning to drive home from the emergency room. Ordinarily, intoxicated patients cannot be legally restrained unless they can be committed under state law, except by police. If a patient is thought to be impaired, it becomes the provider's duty to persuade the patient not to drive, to use a taxi, to call a friend, and as a last resort to contact the police and inform them of the situation. Public safety may take precedence over the patient's right to confidentiality, and failure to notify appropriate authorities of a threat to public safety exposes the physician to liability. This caution may apply especially for employees of the U.S. Department of Transportation. Legal counsel is recommended before notification, as this area is in flux.

Ethical guidelines for physicians and other health care professionals clearly stipulate the responsibility to report an impaired health care provider. The treatment success rate for impaired physicians is among the highest of any patient group. Utilizing intervention services through the licensure board or impaired provider programs allows the impaired provider to maintain professional status, employment, and self-respect by receiving treatment. It also protects the public.

References

1. Bradley K. The primary care practitioner's role in the prevention and management of alcohol problems. Alcohol Health Res World 1994; 18(2):97–104.
2. Barry K, Fleming M. The family physician. Alcohol Health Res World 1994;18(2):105–9.
3. U.S. Department of Health and Human Services. The tenth special report to the U.S. Congress on alcohol and health. Rockville, MD: Public Health Service, National Institutes of Health, National Institute on Alcohol Abuse and Alcoholism, 2000;xiii, 14–17,30,273,283–295,364, 365.
4. Blose J, Holder H. Injury-related medical care utilization in a problem drinking population. Am J Public Health 1991;81:1571–5.
5. American Psychiatric Association. Diagnostic and statistical manual of mental disorders. 3rd rev. ed. Washington, DC: American Psychiatric Press, 1987;173.
6. U.S. Department of Health and Human Services. The seventh special report to the U.S. Congress on alcohol and health. Rockville, MD: Public Health Service, Alcohol, Drug Abuse, and Mental Health Administration, 1990;ix,xv,xxii,xxiv,26,27,33–36,46,119,123,141.

7. Conigliaro J, Maisto SA, McNeil M, et al. Does race make a difference among primary care patients with alcohol problems who agree to enroll in a study of brief interventions? Am J Addict 2000;9(4):321–30.

8. DeWit DJ, Adlaf EA, Offord DR, et al. Age at first alcohol use: a risk factor for the development of alcohol disorders. Am J Psychiatry 2000;157:745–50.

9. Smith D. Social and economic consequences of addiction in America. Commonwealth 1996;90(5):1–4.

10. National Institute on Alcohol Abuse and Alcoholism. Publication no. 35 PH371, January, 1997.

11. Parker DA, Harford TC. Gender-role attitudes, job competition and alcohol consumption among women and men. Alcohol Clin Exp Res 1992;16:159–65.

12. Brower K, Blow F, Beresford T. Treatment implications of chemical dependency models: an integrative approach. J Subst Abuse Treat 1989;6: 147–57.

13. Devor E. A developmental-genetic model of alcoholism: implications for genetic research. J Consult Clin Psychol 1994;62:1108–15.

14. Kaprio J, Viken R, Koskenvuo M, Romanov K, Rose R. Consistency and change in patterns of social drinking: a 6-year follow-up of the Finnish Twin Cohort. Alcohol Clin Exp Res 1992;16:234–40.

15. Wall T, Ehlers C. Acute effects of alcohol on P300 in Asians with different ALDH2 genotypes. Alcohol Clin Exp Res 1995;19:617–22.

16. Kranzler H, Anton R. Implications of recent neuropsychopharmacologic research for understanding the etiology and development of alcoholism. J Consult Clin Psychol 1994;62:1116–26.

17. Schuckit MA, Edenberg HJ, Kalmijn J, et al. A genome-wide search for genes that relate to a low level of response to alcohol. Alcohol Clin Exp Res 2001;25(3):323–9.

18. Goldstein DB. Pharmacology of alcohol. New York: Oxford University Press, 1983;80.

19. Brooks PJ. Brain atrophy and neuronal loss in alcoholism: a role for DNA damage? Neurochem Int 2000;37(5–6):403–12.

20. Maddrey W. Alcoholic hepatitis: clinico-pathologic features and therapy. Semin Liver Dis 1988;8:91–102.

21. Geokas M. Ethanol and the pancreas. Med Clin North Am 1984;68:60–7.

22. Day N, Richardson G. Prenatal alcohol exposure: a continuum of effects. Semin Perinatol 1991;15:272–9.

23. Allen JP, Litten RZ. The role of laboratory tests in alcoholism treatment. J Subst Abuse Treat 2001;81:85.

24. Alexander D, Gwyther R. Alcoholism in adolescents and their families. Pediatr Clin North Am 1995;42:217–30.

25. Allen J, Maisto S, Connors G. Self-report screening tests for alcohol problems in primary care. Arch Intern Med 1995;155:1726–30.

26. Diagnostic and statistical manual of mental disorders, 4th ed. Washington, DC: American Psychiatric Association, 1994;176–83.

27. Connors GJ. Screening for alcohol problems. In: Assessing alcohol problems: a guide for clinicians and researchers. Washington, DC: DHHS, 1995;17–29.

28. Ewing JA. Detecting alcoholism, the CAGE questionnaire. JAMA 1984;252:1905–7.
29. Selzer ML. The Michigan alcoholism screening test: the quest for a new diagnostic instrument. Am J Psychiatry 1971;127:1653–8.
30. U.S. Department of Health and Human Services. Assessing alcohol problem. Rockville, MD: DHHS, 1995: series 4:11, 22, 260. NIH publ. no. 95-3745.
31. Allen JP, Litten RZ, Fertig JB, Babor T. A review of research on the Alcohol Use Disorders Identification Test (AUDIT). Alcohol Clin Exp Res 1997;21(4):613–19.
32. Soyka M, Horak M. Ambulatory detoxification of alcoholic patients—evaluation of a model project (article in German). Gesundheitswesen 2000 Jan;62(1):15–20.
33. Mander A, Young A, Merrick M, et al. Fluid balance, vasopressin and withdrawal symptoms during detoxification from alcohol. Drug Alcohol Depend 1987;24:233–7.
34. Foy A, March S, Drinkwater V. Use of an objective clinical scale in the assessment and management of alcohol withdrawal in a large general hospital. Alcohol Clin Exp Res 1988;12:360–4.
35. Nutt D, Glue P. Neuropharmacological and clinical aspects of alcohol withdrawal. Ann Med 1990;22:275–81.
36. Kramp P, Rafaelsen O. Delirium tremens: a double blind comparison of diazepam and barbital treatment. Acta Psychiatr Scand 1978;58:174–90.
37. Koranyi E, Ravindran A, Seguin J. Alcohol withdrawal concealing symptoms of subdural hematoma—a caveat. Psychiatr J Univ Ottawa 1990;15:15–17.
38. Vaillant G. A summing up: the natural history of alcoholism. Cambridge: Harvard University Press, 1983;307–16.
39. Cross G, Morgan C, Mooney A, Martin C, Rafter J. Alcoholism treatment: a ten-year follow-up study. Alcohol Clin Exp Res 1990;14:169–73.
40. Hoadley J, Fuch B, Holder H. The effect of alcohol beverage restrictions on consumption: a 25 year longitudinal analysis. Am J Drug Alcohol Abuse 1984;10:375–401.
41. O'Malley P, Wagenaar A. Effects of minimum drinking age laws on alcohol use, related behaviors and traffic crash involvement among American youth: 1976–1987. J Stud Alcohol 1991;52:478–91.
42. Jones N, Pieper C, Robertson L. The effect of legal drinking age on fatal injuries of adolescents and young adults. Am J Public Health 1992;82:112–15.
43. Mann R, Vingilis E, Gavin D, Adlaf E, Anglin L. Sentence severity and the drinking driver: relationships with traffic safety outcome. Accid Anal Prev 1991;23:483–91.
44. Green R, French J, Haberman P, Holland P. The effects of combining sanction and rehabilitation for driving under the influence: an evaluation of the New Jersey Countermeasures Program. Accid Anal Prev 1991;23:543–55.

8

Care of the Patient Who Misuses Drugs

Jerome E. Schulz

Patients who misuse drugs are commonly seen by family physicians in the clinic, emergency room, and hospital. Almost all patients who misuse illicit drugs also misuse alcohol and tobacco, and those medical complications are discussed elsewhere in this book (see Chapter 7).

Acute Medical Treatment

Cocaine

Although the illicit use of cocaine declined during the early 1980s, its misuse increased dramatically in 1985 with the marketing of "crack" cocaine. Crack is a highly addictive form of cocaine readily accessible at a low cost (as inexpensive as $5 to $10). Crack cocaine misuse has changed cocaine from a drug of the rich and affluent to a drug anyone can afford (including adolescents and children). Cocaine continues to be one of the most commonly reported illicit drugs causing emergency room visits. The age of the average cocaine user has dropped substantially, and the number of female cocaine abusers has risen since the mid-1980s. The use of cocaine has declined over the past 5 years.

Cocaine hydrochloride is water-soluble and can be injected intravenously or inhaled intranasally (snorted). Cocaine hydrochloride cannot be smoked because it decomposes. If it is dissolved in ether and distilled, the base form of cocaine (freebase) is reprecipitated, and this substance can be smoked. "Crack" cocaine is produced by dissolving cocaine hydrochloride in sodium bicarbonate and distilling off the water. It then forms "rocks," which can be smoked. The term *crack* comes from the noise the rocks make as they are heated and smoked.

Effects

Cocaine causes euphoria, talkativeness, increased energy, and increased confidence. Rapid euphoria is followed by a letdown characterized by depression, irritability, restlessness, and a generalized feeling of uneasiness and discomfort. When misusers start feeling letdown, they use more cocaine, which results in blood levels that frequently cause medical complications and can be lethal. Alcohol is frequently used with cocaine and forms cocaethylene, which produces prolonged symptoms and toxicity.[1] The most frequent presenting complaints for patients misusing cocaine are listed in Table 8.1. Physical findings suggestive of cocaine misuse include agitation, dehydration, malnutrition, tachycardia, elevated blood pressure, rhinorrhea, singed eyebrows (from crack or freebase smoking), coughing, wheezing, poor dentition, and a generally unkempt appearance.

Complications

The three primary cardiovascular complications of cocaine abuse are hypertension, myocardial ischemia, and cardiac arrhythmias. Cardiac toxicity can occur with all three routes of administration (intranasal, intravenous, and inhaled). In individuals who are sensitive to cocaine or who have coronary artery disease, cardiac symptoms can occur with relatively low doses of cocaine. Cocaine's effect on the heart

Table 8.1. **Chief Complaints and Presenting Problems—Cocaine**

Chest pain
Cardiac arrhythmias
New-onset seizures
Recurrent sinusitis
Anxiety problems
Cough
Chronic nasal problems
Headache
Sleep disorders
Family dysfunction
Weight loss
Obstetrical complications

appears to be caused by blocking the reuptake of norepinephrine at the neuronal synapses. The norepinephrine excess produces an increased heart rate and increased blood pressure; simultaneous coronary vasospasm decreases the myocardial oxygen supply. The increased cardiac work load with decreased oxygenation causes chest pains in one half to two thirds of heavy cocaine users. Cocaine also enhances platelet aggregation and in situ thrombus formation.[2]

Hypertension usually responds to diazepam 5 to 10 mg IV repeated for three doses if needed.[3] If the blood pressure does not respond, give an α-adrenergic blocker such as phentolamine, or a direct vasodilator such as nitrates, hydralazine, or nitroprusside intravenously.[4] Beta-blocking agents should not be used because in conjunction with cocaine they increase vasoconstriction, increase the blood pressure, decrease left ventricular function, and can cause a paroxysmal increase in heart rate.

Cocaine causes myocardial ischemia and chest pain (see Chapter 76). Cocaine misuse should be suspected in any young patient who presents with chest pain. The risk of an acute myo-cardial infarction increases dramatically after the use of cocaine.[5] A positive urine drug screen for benzoylecgonine (a metabolite of cocaine) confirms the presence of cocaine.

Electrocardiographic (ECG) changes of ischemia are common, but occasionally are not present even with an acute myocardial infarction caused by cocaine. It is impossible to clinically differentiate patients with cocaine-induced chest pain and those experiencing a myocardial infarction.[6] Patients frequently do not admit they have been using cocaine.[7] If patients are "coming down" from a cocaine binge, they may have significant chest pain but do not report it.[8]

The evaluation of cocaine misusers with chest pain is also complicated by increased serum creatine kinase containing M and B subunits caused by cocaine-induced rhabdomyolysis.[9] Cardiac troponin I is more specific for the diagnosis of myocardial infarction in patients with cocaine-associated ischemia.

Nitroglycerin relieves the coronary spasm caused by cocaine, and it should be used as the initial treatment.[10] Phentolamine can be used if the chest pain persists. Thrombolytic therapy appears to be safe for cocaine-associated myocardial infarction after the blood pressure is normal unless a subarachnoid hemorrhage or aortic dissection is suspected.[11] Calcium channel blocking agents should be used cautiously because animal studies have shown they increase cocaine's cardiac toxicity. Patients with cocaine-induced myocardial infarction should not be treated with beta-blocking agents. Chronic cocaine misuse causes myocardial fibrosis and congestive heart failure.[12]

The most common arrhythmia associated with cocaine misuse is tachycardia, but it usually resolves spontaneously as the drug is metabolized or with use of an anxiolytic agent. Cocaine-induced wide complex dysrhythmias associated with acidosis need to be treated aggressively with sodium bicarbonate.[13] Both acidosis and hyperthermia (which should be treated aggressively with rapid cooling to prevent rhabdomyolysis and subsequent renal failure) are associated with a poor prognosis in cocaine intoxication.[14] Because cocaine has properties similar to those of type I antiarrhythmic agents (procainamide and quinidine), the potential exists for increased toxicity if these agents are used to treat cocaine-induced arrhythmias.[15] If patients state that they have a feeling of "impending doom," cardiovascular collapse may be imminent. Initial euphoria rapidly changes to irritability with hallucinations. After an initial elevation of the pulse and blood pressure, the patient may experience a rapid fall in blood pressure and develop life-threatening cardiac arrhythmias. Other cardiovascular complications caused by cocaine misuse are aortic rupture, subacute and acute endocarditis (for injection drug users), pneumopericardium, and left ventricular hypertrophy.

Smugglers may swallow large bags of cocaine to prevent detection ("body packing"). Rupture of the bags causes severe cocaine intoxication, which can be treated with activated charcoal (50–100 g in adults) and a cathartic along with all the treatments described above. The term *body stuffing* describes the ingestion of cocaine packets to hide the evidence when confronted by the police. This usually involves lesser quantities of cocaine but it can lead to more toxicity because the cocaine is poorly wrapped. Frequently it does not show up on x-ray.[16]

Seizures are common with cocaine misuse. Cocaine decreases the seizure threshold and increases the body temperature, which makes an individual more susceptible to seizures. The increased body temperature is caused by vasoconstriction and increased muscle activity. Seizures may also be a terminal event in severe overdose patients. Children passively exposed to cocaine in crack houses or small confined areas where crack is being smoked may have seizures. Cocaine and cocaethylene can also be ingested by breastfeeding infants. A urine toxicology screen for benzoylecgonine should be considered for all children presenting with their first seizure.[17] Intravenous diazepam is the treatment of choice for seizures caused by cocaine.

Subarachnoid hemorrhages occur with cocaine misuse. They are caused by ruptured aneurysms or arteriovenous malformations secondary to the marked elevation in the blood pressure from cocaine.

Cerebral infarction associated with cocaine misuse may be caused by vasoconstriction and increased platelet aggregation caused by cocaine. A urine toxicology screen should be obtained on any young person presenting with stroke symptoms. There are reported cases of cerebral infarction in infants born to mothers who misused cocaine during pregnancy.[18] Cocaine misuse should be considered in patients who have a sudden onset of severe new headaches, which may precede a cerebral vascular accident.

Serious obstetric complications, including abruptio placentae, spontaneous abortions, premature labor, and stillbirths, are increased in cocaine-misusing pregnant women.[19] Intrauterine exposure to cocaine causes fetal atrial and ventricular arrhythmias, congestive heart failure, cardiorespiratory arrest, and fetal death.[20] Newborn infants may demonstrate signs of cocaine withdrawal, including irritability, tremulousness, and poor eating. Maternal–infant bonding is poor. Although long-term effects are not clear, cocaine babies may have developmental delays and attention-deficit disorders.[21]

The most common psychiatric symptoms of cocaine misuse are paranoia, anxiety, and depression. Paranoia occurs in 80% to 90% of heavy cocaine misusers, and these patients are at high risk to develop a psychosis. The psychosis (similar to an amphetamine psychosis) may seem to be an acute schizophrenic episode, but it clears within 12 to 24 hours. Hallucinations called "snow lights" (flashing visual hallucinations) and "coke bugs" (tactile and visual hallucinations) are common with cocaine misuse. Patients experience withdrawal symptoms when they stop using cocaine. Initially, they become lethargic and somnolent. Depression is common after cocaine cessation, and patients frequently experience severe anhedonia that may last several months (antidepressants such as desipramine may help).

Smoking cocaine can cause a cough with black sputum production and dyspnea. Hemoptysis and spontaneous pneumothorax are common in crack addicts. Pulmonary edema (noncardiac) may be an acute hypersensitivity reaction. Patients with "crack lung syndrome" have fever, marked bronchospasm, infiltrates, eosinophilia, marked pruritus, and increased immunoglobulin E (IgE). Bronchiolitis obliterans and organizing pneumonia (BOOP) has been reported in crack cocaine users. Both crack lung and BOOP may respond to high-dose systemic steroids.[22] Asthma can be exacerbated by smoking crack cocaine. Pollutants in crack can also cause bronchitis and tracheitis.

Severe rhabdomyolysis is rare, but mild cases are seen in one third of the patients seen in emergency rooms for cocaine overdoses. In severe cases, 15% of patients die with renal hepatic failure and disseminated intravascular coagulation.[23] The prognosis worsens with increased temperature, seizures, and hypotension. Rhabdomyolysis is an acute medical emergency and requires intensive treatment to prevent death. Initial treatment should focus on preventing renal damage and establishing diuresis. Hyperthermia should be treated aggressively with cooling to prevent rhabdomyolysis. Muscle activity should be decreased and seizures prevented to limit rhabdomyolysis.

Almost all patients who snort cocaine have chronic sinusitis. They may have unilateral inflammation of the nose (cocaine addicts frequently snort in one nostril at a time so only one nostril is inflamed). Chronic rhinitis, perforations of the nasal septum, and abscessed teeth are common in cocaine snorters. Patients who misuse cocaine frequently engage in high-risk sexual behaviors that expose them to sexually transmitted diseases and human immunodeficiency virus (HIV) disease.

Opiate Intoxication

Heroin is the most commonly misused opiate. Over the past 10 years, emergency room (ER) visits due to heroin overdose have dramatically increased. The 2000 DAWN survey showed the largest increase in 12- to 17-year-old youths in whom ER visits have quadrupled.[24] In the 1999 Household Inventory Survey, 2.3% of eighth graders had used heroin at some time in their lives. Most new heroin abusers are snorting and smoking the drug. Recently the abuse of OxyContin has reached epidemic levels. Opiate overdoses occur in new users, in older users who have stopped using and lost their drug tolerance, whenever the purity of the street drug increases, and whenever a more potent opiate (e.g., fentanyl) is substituted for heroin. The recent purity of the drug has increased and the average price has decreased by two thirds. Before the drug is sold on the streets, pure heroin is adulterated (cut) with quinine, lactose, mannitol, dextrose, or talc, and will sell for as little as $10 (a dime bag). A history of heroin abuse is usually available from patients, their friends or family, or the hospital record.

The presenting signs and symptoms of opiate overdose are stupor, miosis, hypotension, bradycardia, and decreased bowel sounds. Frequently needle marks or tracks are present. In more severe cases, respiratory depression with apnea and pulmonary edema can occur. Seizures are seen with meperidine and propoxyphene overdoses. A urine toxicology screen detects most opiates except fentanyl.

Naloxone (Narcan) is the primary treatment for opiate overdose. An initial intravenous dose of 0.4 to 0.8 mg usually reverses the opiate effects. This dose can be repeated every 2 to 3 minutes up to a total dose of 10 to 20 mg. The goal in treatment is to reverse the respiratory depression, not to get the patient awake and alert, which may precipitate an acute withdrawal syndrome and make the patient hostile and potentially violent. Higher doses of naloxone are needed for codeine, propoxyphene, and pentazocine overdoses. Patients with pulmonary edema should be intubated. Positive end-expiratory pressure ventilation is used if necessary. Diuretics and digitalis are not effective therapies to treat opiate-induced pulmonary edema. In high dosages, naloxone has been reported to cause pulmonary edema, convulsions, and asystole in about 1% of treated patients.[25] The half-life of naloxone is shorter than that of most opiates, so patients may need to be treated with repeated doses of naloxone. For propoxyphene and methadone overdoses, an intravenous drip of naloxone (0.2–0.8 mg/h) can be used. Some authors advocate discharging heroin overdose patients without hospital admission if they are stable (usually after 8–12 hours of observation).[26] Patients who have attempted suicide, used other potentiating drugs, or for whom there is a question about the opiate used should be admitted for observation.

Pregnant heroin addicts or pregnant patients on methadone present a special problem. Because there is an increased risk of serious complications to the fetus, pregnant women should not be withdrawn from opiates. They should be maintained on methadone through the pregnancy. Hyperactivity, irritability, hyperreflexia, yawning, tachypnea, tremors and myoclonic seizures, poor sleep patterns, vomiting, and diarrhea characterize the neonatal withdrawal syndrome. Every attempt should be made to modify the infant's environment to reduce external stimuli. Phenobarbital and paregoric are used to treat withdrawing newborns.[27]

In the future, family physicians may be allowed to provide long-term maintenance therapy (methadone and buprenorphine) to heroin addicts.[28]

Amphetamines

Emergency room visits for amphetamine misuse have increased. The introduction of "ice" to the drug scene may account for this increase. Ice (Hawaiian ice) is methamphetamine made in the Far East and smuggled through Hawaii into the continental United States. *Crack* and *crank* are two street terms that are commonly confused. Crank is a street name for methamphetamine that can be taken as pills, injected, or snorted. Crack is freebase cocaine. The effects and complications of amphetamine misuse are similar to those of cocaine except amphetamines have a longer half-life.

Agitation is the most common presenting symptom of amphetamine misuse. Hallucinations, suicidal ideation, delusions, and confusion may be present. Cardiac symptoms include chest pain, palpitations, and myocardial infarction. Intracranial hemorrhagic strokes in young patients (15–45 years old) are associated with amphetamine abuse.[29] Acute signs of amphetamine intoxication include an elevation in the blood pressure and pulse, dilated pupils, tremor, cardiac arrhythmias, and increased reflexes. The long-term effects of amphetamine abuse include impaired concentration, abrupt mood changes, weight loss, paranoid delusions, and violence. Amphetamine psychosis is a combination of paranoid delusions with hallucinations; it can be treated with benzodiazepines.

Marijuana

Marijuana is the most commonly abused illicit drug. Its use has recently increased in adolescents, and the perception of marijuana's harmful effects has decreased.[30] In the 1999 National Institute of Drug Abuse (NIDA) Household Survey, which is available through the NIDA Web site, an estimated 14.8 million people (6.7% of the population) used marijuana in the month prior to the interview. Marijuana is a mixture of compounds, with the most psychoactive being Δ9-tetrahydrocannabinol (THC). Hashish, which is more potent than regular marijuana, refers to a dried resin made from the flower tops of the cannabis plant. Sinsemilla is a seedless form of marijuana that is approximately twice as potent as hashish. Marijuana is smoked in "joints," "bowls" (miniature pipes), or "bongs" (water- or air-cooled smoking devices that enable the smoker to inhale more drug with less irritation). Marijuana smoke has a pungent odor that can be identified on the clothes of chronic marijuana misusers.

Patients smoke marijuana to achieve a state of euphoria and relaxation. Users become less inhibited and laugh spontaneously. Marijuana may be "laced" with other drugs, such as cocaine, phencyclidine (PCP), or other hallucinogens, causing bizarre reactions. Marijuana is highly lipophilic, with a half-life of approximately 3 days. Impaired concentration, judgment, and coordination can last up to 2 days after using marijuana.

Chronic marijuana smoking leads to dependence with increased tolerance and withdrawal symptoms when the drug is stopped. Withdrawal symptoms include irritability, drowsiness, increased sleeping, and increased intake of high carbohydrate foods ("marijuana munchies"). Depression, paranoia, and anxiety are common effects of chronic marijuana misuse. Long-term abuse of marijuana may cause permanent cognitive impairment especially in patients who start abusing the drug at a young age.[31] Marijuana may impair the immune system and promote tumor growth,[32] a particularly important point when caring for HIV-positive patients.

The most common physical signs of marijuana misuse are tachycardia and conjunctival irritation (which may be masked in experienced users by using eyedrops). Urine testing is the most effective laboratory method for screening patients suspected of marijuana misuse. In daily misusers, urine toxicology screens may remain positive for several weeks. After a single misuse episode the urine test is positive for 3 to 4 days. When an adolescent is experiencing deterioration in school performance or a marked change in personality or behavior, a urine drug screen for marijuana should be done before formal psychological or psychiatric testing.

Designer/Club Drugs

Designer drugs are compounds that are chemically altered derivatives of federally controlled substances. They are changed slightly to produce special mood-altering effects. Contaminant by-products cause many of the complications of designer drugs produced in basement laboratories. The best known designer drug is ecstasy (3,4-methylenedioxymethamphetamine, MDMA), which is commonly used at "rave" parties. MDMA's use by teenagers has increased significantly in the past 5 years.[33] MDMA, which is ingested orally, causes euphoria, increased self-esteem, enhanced communication skills, and an elevated mood. Adverse effects include jaw clenching, tachycardia, panic attacks, nausea and vomiting, nystagmus, inhibited ejaculation, and urinary urgency. The letdown after taking MDMA, which lasts 1 to 3 days, is characterized by drowsiness, muscle aches, jaw soreness, depression, and difficulty concentrating. As more of the drug is ingested, the toxic effects increase and the euphoric effects decrease. Recent evidence shows that chronic MDMA abuse can cause permanent brain damage.[34]

Other commonly abused club drugs are γ-hydroxybutyric acid (GHB), flunitrazepam (Rohypnol), and ketamine. GHB is used primarily by adolescents and young adults at nightclubs or raves and by body builders as a muscle builder. Emergency room mentions of GHB increased from 55 in 1994 to 2,973 in 1999.[24] It is usually combined with alcohol to cause relaxation, intoxication and euphoria.[35] It has increasingly been involved in overdoses causing severe respiratory depression and death. Withdrawal symptoms occur and GHB is one of the "date rapes" drugs because it causes amnesia. GHB's effect is short acting (about 4 hours) and overdoses can be treated with respiratory support.

Ketamine (Special K, Vitamin K and K) is an anesthetic that causes a dream-like state, loss of inhibitions, and hallucinations. It can be injected, snorted, or smoked with marijuana. In high doses it causes delirium, amnesia (making it another "date rape" drug), elevated blood pressure, depression, and potentially fatal respiratory depression. Rohypnol (roofies, rophies, roche, or the forget-me pill), the third "date rape" drug,[36] is a benzodiazepine used in Europe and Latin America as a sedative/hypnotic. It is usually ingested orally with alcohol. Rohypnol has a long half-life, so overdoses need prolonged respiratory support. Flumazenil (a benzodiazepine antagonist) has been used in severe overdose patients (0.02 mg/kg in children and 0.2 mg in adults and repeat 0.3 mg up to a total dose of 3 mg).

Hallucinogens

Hallucinogens are defined as drugs that produce visual, auditory, tactile, and in some cases olfactory hallucinations. Lysergic acid diethylamide (LSD) is the most potent, most common hallucinogen. It is referred to as acid, dots, cubes, window pane, or blotter. LSD can cause bizarre behavior that begins a few minutes after ingestion, peaks in about 3 to 4 hours, and lasts up to 12 hours. Paranoia, depression, anxiety, acute psychosis, combative behavior, and panic attacks are associated with "bad trips." Patients experiencing adverse reactions to hallucinogens can be confused with patients having a schizophrenic reaction. Patients toxic from hallucinogens (1) have no history of mental illness, (2) tell you they have ingested the drug, and (3) have visual instead of auditory hallucinations. On physical examination, patients have pronounced pupillary dilation, tachycardia, sweating, and fever. Patients diagnosed with LSD intoxication need to be carefully screened for other problems such as hypoglycemia, head trauma, drug withdrawal, electrolyte abnormalities, endocrine disease, central nervous system (CNS) infection, hypoxia, and toxic reactions to other street or prescription drugs. Frequently patients can be "talked down" in a quiet setting. If necessary for severe agitation, a benzodiazepine can be used.[38] Patients may have chronic effects from LSD that include flashbacks, psychoses, depressive reactions, and chronic personality changes.

Phencyclidine

The complications of phencyclidine (PCP) misuse are still seen in emergency rooms. PCP intoxication is a frequently missed diagnosis, and physicians must be aware of the potential toxicity of PCP and its presenting signs and symptoms. PCP can be an adulterant, and patients may not know they took the drug. PCP can be smoked with cocaine (space-basing). In low doses PCP causes euphoria and sedation. Increasing doses can cause hypertension, muscle rigidity, seizures, and coma. The presence of nystagmus, rapidly changing behaviors, and muscle rigidity help distinguish PCP intoxication from stimulant and hallucinogen overdoses. A urine drug screen helps diagnose PCP intoxication.

The treatment of PCP intoxication depends on the stage of intoxication. Mild intoxication can be treated with quiet observation and a benzodiazepine for combative behavior. Benadryl can be given for dystonic reactions. Physical restraints should be avoided because they increase the risk of rhabdomyolysis. Activated charcoal helps eliminate the drug and prevents reabsorption. Propranolol can be given intravenously for severe hypertension and tachycardia (contraindicated if the patient has used cocaine with PCP). Patients should be catheterized to prevent urine retention. Furosemide (Lasix) can increase urine flow and PCP excretion. The toxic effects of PCP can last up to 24 hours.

Volatile Substances

Volatile substance misuse (gasoline, airplane glue, cleaning agents, Freon, typewriter fluid, and lighter fluid) is common among early adolescent boys in large urban areas and on North American Indian reservations.[39] The agents are used to "get high," and they cause euphoria, light-headedness, a state of excitation, and frequently hallucinations. They are inexpensive and readily available. Volatile substances are sniffed, "bagged" (inhaling the substance from a plastic or paper bag), and "huffed" (inhaling the vapors by holding a piece of cloth soaked in the volatile substance against the mouth and nose).

Volatile substances are rapidly absorbed into the bloodstream, are highly lipid-soluble, and produce marked CNS effects (depression most commonly). They frequently cause nausea and vomiting. Tolerance and dependence (with withdrawal symptoms) can develop. In the emergency room, solvent misuse frequently can be mistaken for acute psychiatric problems because of the altered mental state and hallucinations. Solvent abuse should be suspected in teenagers who suddenly collapse while partying. Chronic abuse causes permanent damage to the brain (toluene), liver (chlorinated hydrocarbons, chloroform, trichloroethane, and trichloroethylene), heart, kidneys, and bone marrow (benzene).

Airplane glue causes peripheral neuropathies, tremors, and ataxia. Gasoline causes coughing and wheezing secondary to irritation to the respiratory tract and frequently intense hallucinations. Anemia, cardiac arrhythmias, and confusion are also seen with gasoline intoxication, and renal toxicity can be detected by proteinuria. Freon is cardiotoxic and causes arrhythmias. Typewriter fluid (trichloroethylene) causes neuropathies, headache, cardiac arrhythmias, renal and hepatic dysfunction, and diffuse CNS symptoms.

When teenagers present with confusion, physicians must be sensitive to the smell of solvents on the clothes or breath of patients. Unusual burns are indicative of solvent abuse. Laboratory tests may show an abnormal blood count, and urinalysis may reveal protein or blood in the urine. Liver function tests may be elevated. With chronic solvent abuse, the chest radiograph may reveal an enlarged heart. Supportive care for acute inhalant toxicity usually allows symptoms to clear within 4 to 6 hours. Benzodiazepines are indicated for seizures, and haloperidol (Haldol) can be used for extreme agitation. Cardiac monitoring is frequently necessary.

Care of Patients in Recovery

Overview

Little has been written about the care of patients after they recover from drug and alcohol addiction. Because many medical problems resolve as patients abstain from illicit drugs and alcohol, it is reasonable to wait a few months before treating less severe medical problems. Patients in recovery must be screened to ensure their continued abstinence from drugs and alcohol. A few brief questions can help with the assessment (Table 8.2). Patients in active recovery programs answer these questions in a straightforward manner. If family members are present, ask them how the patient is doing. Positive support of patients, even if they have relapsed, is imperative. Physicians should emphasize the need to have accurate current drug misuse information to prevent serious side effects with prescription medications.

Table 8.2. **Recovery Assessment Questions**

Are you attending aftercare or recovery meetings?
When was the last time you attended a meeting?
Do you have a sponsor, and when did you last contact him or her?
What step are you working on (if patient is in a 12-step program)?

Any medication has the potential to cause a relapse, especially mood-altering medications. Prescription medications can cause a relapse by lowering patients' resistance or by patients becoming addicted to the prescribed medication. The following guidelines are for patients with a history of drug and alcohol addiction[40]:

1. Whenever possible, use nonpharmacologic treatments. Encourage patients to exercise, meditate, and change their diet; use acupuncture or biofeedback before prescribing medications.
2. Avoid benzodiazepines and narcotics. If they are necessary, patients should be carefully monitored with regularly scheduled follow-up visits.
3. Be cautious about prescribing "cue stimuli" medications, such as inhalants in former intranasal cocaine addicts.
4. Use "alternate" drugs, such as antidepressants for chronic pain or buspirone (BuSpar) for anxiety, because they have less addiction potential.
5. Choose medications with side effects that may be beneficial, such as beta-blocking drugs to treat hypertension because they decrease anxiety, which is common during early recovery.
6. Beware of increased drug sensitivity secondary to damage caused by patients' previous drug and alcohol misuse. Patients need a thorough evaluation focusing on specific complications from their previous addiction. Injection drug users must be assessed for hepatitis and HIV disease.
7. Before prescribing medications, wait for normal resolution of medical problems associated with withdrawal and early recovery, such as hypertension, depression, hyperglycemia and tachycardia.
8. Anticipate the normal changes (insomnia, anxiety, depression, and some sexual dysfunction) that occur during recovery and counsel patients about them so the patients are less likely to be concerned or to seek medications.

Treatment of Specific Diseases

The treatment of many common diseases can be complicated in patients with a history of drug/alcohol addiction. Most injection drug abusers have HIV disease (up to 90% in some areas) and frequently they abuse alcohol. Antiviral drugs that cause liver or pancreatic problems need to be avoided or used very cautiously. The dose of methadone in methadone maintenance patients may have to be altered after beginning antiviral therapy. Several antiviral drugs have side effects that mimic the narcotic withdrawal syndrome, making it difficult to differentiate drug side effects from narcotic withdrawal. Ritonavir formulations contain alcohol and cause a severe reaction in patients taking disulfiram. The alcohol may cause a relapse.

In managing acute and chronic pain in patients in recovery, every effort should be made to avoid narcotic medications by using nonsteroidal antiinflammatory drugs. If narcotics are needed, they should be prescribed for a limited period and with a fixed-dose schedule instead of "as needed."

Medications for upper respiratory infections frequently contain drugs that can jeopardize patients in recovery. Most cough syrups contain alcohol and codeine, and they should be avoided in patients in recovery. Several over-the-counter cough suppressants are available that do not contain alcohol. Pseudoephedrine is a stimulant, and it is potentially dangerous in former cocaine addicts.

Care of Patients Who Continue to Misuse Drugs

Treating patients for any medical problem while they misuse drugs and alcohol is difficult. The primary goal should be to help patients with their drug and alcohol misuse. A physician's caring nonjudgmental recommendation to abstain can be effective, especially if the recommendation is connected to the patient's present medical problem. Studies have shown that brief interventions by primary care physicians can decrease alcohol consumption.[41] Patients should be encouraged to enter a drug and alcohol treatment program. Most patients can be treated as outpatients unless they have significant medical or psychiatric problems. Detoxification may require a brief hospitalization. If a physician is uncomfortable treating patients who continue to misuse drugs, patients should be referred to another physician. To prevent a serious or potentially fatal reaction caused by concurrent drug or alcohol misuse, physicians must be extremely cautious when prescribing any medication to patients misusing drugs or alcohol. Poor medication compliance is a major problem with patients who continue to misuse drugs and alcohol.

References

1. Farre M, De La Torre R, Gonzalez M, Roset PN, Menoyo E, Cami J. Cocaine and alcohol interactions in humans: neuroendocrine effects and cocaethylene metabolism. J Pharmacol Exp Ther 1997;283:164–76.

2. Heesch CM, Wilhelm CR, Ristic J, Adnane J, Bontepo FA, Wagner WR. Cocaine activates platelets and increases the formation of circulating platelet containing microaggregates in humans. Heart 2000;83:688–95.
3. Goldfrank LR, Hoffman RS. The cardiovascular effects of cocaine. Ann Emerg Med 1991;20:165–75.
4. Nolan AG. Recreational drug misuse: issues for the cardiologist. Heart 2000;83:627–33.
5. Mittleman MA, Mintzer D, Maclure M, Tofler GH, Sherwood JB, Muller JE. Triggering of myocardial infarction by cocaine. Circulation 1999;99:2737–41.
6. Hollander JE, Hoffman RS, Gennis P, et al. Prospective multicenter evaluation of cocaine-associated chest pain. Acad Emerg Med 1994;1:330–9.
7. McNagny SD, Parker RM. High prevalence of recent cocaine use and the unreliability of patient self-report in an inner-city walk-in clinic. JAMA 1992;267:1106–8.
8. Trabulsy ME. Cocaine washed out syndrome in a patient with acute myocardial infarction. Am J Emerg Med 1995;13:538–9.
9. Rubin RB, Neugarten J. Cocaine-induced rhabdomyolysis masquerading as myocardial ischemia. Am J Med 1989;86:551–3.
10. Brogan WC, Lange RA, Kim AS, Moliterno DJ, Hillis LD. Alleviation of cocaine-induced coronary vasoconstriction by nitroglycerin. J Am Coll Cardiol 1991;18:581–6.
11. Hollander JE, Burstein JL, Hoffman RS, Shih RD, Wilson LD. Cocaine-associated myocardial infarction. Chest 1995;107:1237–41.
12. Hogya PT, Wolfson AB. Chronic cocaine abuse associated with dilated cardiomyopathy. Am J Emerg Med 1991;8:203–4.
13. Kerns W, Garvey L, Owens J. Cocaine-induced wide complex dysrhythmia. J Emerg Med 1997;15(3):321–9.
14. Stevens DC, Campbell JP, Carter JE, Waston WA. Acid-base abnormalities associated with cocaine toxicity in emergency department patients. Clin Toxicol 1994;32:31–9.
15. Om A, Ellahham S, DiSciascio G. Management of cocaine-induced cardiovascular complications. Am Heart J 1993;125:469–75.
16. June R, Aks SE, Keys N, Wahl M. Medical outcome of cocaine bodystuffers. J Emerg Med 2000;18(2):221–4.
17. Mott SH, Packer RJ, Soldin SJ. Neurologic manifestations of cocaine exposure in childhood. Pediatrics 1994;93:557–60.
18. Chasnoff IJ, Bussey ME, Savich R, Stack CM. Perinatal cerebral infarction and maternal cocaine use. J Pediatr 1986;108:456–9.
19. Cohen HR, Green JR, Crombleholm WR. Peripartum cocaine use: estimating risk of adverse pregnancy outcome. Int J Gynecol Obstet 1991; 35:51–4.
20. Frassica JJ, Orav EJ, Walsh EP, Lipshultz SE. Arrhythmias in children prenatally exposed to cocaine. Arch Pediatr Adolesc Med 1994;148: 1163–9.
21. Arendt R, Angelopoulos J, Salvator A, Singer L. Motor development of cocaine-exposed children at age two years. Pediatrics 1999;103:86–92.
22. Haim DY, Lippmann ML, Goldberg SK, Walkenstein MD. The pulmonary complications of crack cocaine. Chest 1995;107:233–49.

23. Roth D, Alarcon FJ, Fernandez JA, Preston RA, Bourgoignie JJ. Acute rhabdomyolysis associated with cocaine intoxication. N Engl J Med 1988;319:673–7.
24. DAWN Report 2000. Substance Abuse and Mental Health Services Administration. Available at *www.samhsa.gov*.
25. Osterwalder JJ. Naloxone—for intoxication with intravenous heroin and heroin mixtures—harmless of hazardous? J Toxicol Clin Toxicol 1996; 34(4):409–16.
26. Smith DA, Leake L, Loflin JR, Yealy DM. Is admission after intravenous heroin overdose necessary? Ann Emerg Med 1992;21:1326–30.
27. Levy M, Spino M. Neonatal withdrawal syndrome: associated drugs and pharmacological management. Pharmacotherapy 1993;13:202–11.
28. O'Connor PG, Fiellin DA. Pharmacologic treatment of heroin-dependent patients. Ann Intern Med 2000;133:40–54.
29. Buxton N, McConachie NS. Amphetamine abuse and intracranial haemorrhage. J R Soc Med 2000;93:472–7.
30. Mathias R. Student's use of marijuana, other illicit drugs, and cigarettes continued to rise in 1995. NIDA Notes 1996;Jan/Feb. Vol III(1). Available online http://165.112.61/NIDAHome.html under NIDA Notes Newsletter.
31. Solwij N. Do cognitive impairments recover following cessation of cannabis use? Life Sci 1995;56:2119–26.
32. Zhu LX, Sharma S, Stolina M, et al. Delta-9-tetrahydrocannabinol inhibits antitumor immunity by a CB2 receptor-mediated, cytokine dependent pathway. J Immunol 2000;165(1):373–80.
33. Zickler P. Annual survey finds increasing teen use of ecstasy, steroids. NIDA Notes 2001;16(2). Available online http://165.112.61/NIDA-Home.html under NIDA Notes Newsletter.
34. Statement of the director of the National Institute of Drug Abuse. U.S. Senate caucus on international narcotics control. Available at *www.drugabuse.gov/Testimony/7-25-00Testimony.html*.
35. Nicholson KL, Balster RL. GHB: a new and novel drug of abuse. Drug Alcohol Depend 2001;63:1–22.
36. Waltzman ML. Flunitrazepam: A review of "roofies". Pediatr Emerg Care 1999;15(1):59–60.
37. Nicholson KL, Balster RL. GHB: a new and novel drug of abuse. Drug Alcohol Depend 2001;63:1–22.
38. Blaho K, Merigian K, Winbery S, Geraci SA, Smartt C. Clinical pharmacology of lysergic acid diethylamine: case reports and review of the treatment of intoxication. Am J Ther 1997;4:211–21.
39. Kurtzman TL, Otsuka K, Wahl R. Inhalant abuse by adolescents. J Adolesc Health 2001;28:170–80.
40. Schulz JE. The integration of medical management with recovery. J Psychoactive Drugs 1997;29(3):233–7.
41. Fleming MF, Barry RL, Manwell LB, Johnson, London R. Brief physicians' advice for problem alcohol drinkers: a randomized controlled trial in community based primary care practice. JAMA 1997;277:1039–45.

9
Care of the Patient with Chronic Pain

Carole Nistler

Chronic pain is pain that persists beyond the usual healing time for tissue injury. It is often defined as pain lasting longer than 3 to 6 months.[1-3] It may or may not represent continuing tissue pathology. Family physicians encounter many nonmalignant disease states that involve chronic pain, such as headache, trigeminal neuralgia, neck injury, low back problems, arthritis, and peripheral neuropathy.

The management of chronic pain is challenging because a patient's symptoms may not be confirmed by physical examinations, laboratory tests, or diagnostic procedures. Chronic pain represents a complex interaction of physical, psychological, social, and spiritual factors.

Physiology of Pain and Pain Management

The experience of pain is initiated by stimulation of nociceptors located in skin, subcutaneous tissue, viscera, muscle, periosteum, joints, and so on. Interneurons located in the dorsal horn of the spinal cord control whether impulses transmitted from the nociceptors are subsequently transmitted to the rest of the central nervous system (CNS). Interference with pain transmission at the level of the interneuron in the dorsal horn may explain the effectiveness of peripheral stimuli in modifying pain perception, e.g., massage, acupuncture, transcutaneous external nerve stimulation (TENS), and capsaicin cream.

Descending control of the pain response from the CNS can be activated by arousal, attention, and emotional stress, and, via descending pathways and receptors, they can also modify the pain experience. CNS modification of pain transmission explains the effectiveness of cognitive-behavioral therapies such as biofeedback training, visualization, and music therapy.[2,4]

The action of specific neurotransmitters involved in CNS control of pain perception can be modified by a growing number of adjunctive agents used in pain management. Baclofen (Lioresal), benzodiazepines, and the many antiepileptic drugs such as carbamazepine (Tegretol) work by binding to γ-aminobutyric acid (GABA) receptors in the dorsal horn.[4]

Opioid analgesics modulate the pain response by binding to opioid receptors located in the dorsal horn and other areas of the spinal cord and brain. Opioid receptors are classified as mu, kappa, or sigma. Opioid drugs that bind primarily to mu-opioid receptors produce analgesia, euphoria, respiratory depression, and bradycardia. These agents are known as mu-opioids or pure mu-agonists and include codeine, hydrocodone, morphine, oxycodone, and hydromorphone. Opioids of the agonist-antagonist type have a primarily kappa-agonist analgesic effect, but a mu-receptor antagonist effect, thereby producing limited analgesia.[4,5]

The physiology underlying the use of nonsteroidal antiinflammatory drugs (NSAIDs) for pain control relate to their ability to inhibit prostaglandin synthesis at sites of tissue injury. This produces both an analgesic and antiinflammatory effect. NSAIDs act on the cyclooxygenase (COX) enzyme system that produces prostaglandins. COX enzymes are classified into two isoforms—COX-1 isoforms found in the gastrointestinal tract, renal tract, and platelets, and COX-2 sites found in areas of inflammation and in the CNS. Selective COX-2 inhibitor drugs have been developed to provide the analgesic benefit of an NSAID with fewer gastrointestinal and bleeding diathesis side effects.[6]

Therapeutic Choices

The World Health Organization (WHO)[7] has promoted a three-step approach to cancer pain management that is also widely recommended and used for chronic noncancer pain.[2,8] The WHO approach recommends first the use of nonopioid drugs starting with acetaminophen and then the NSAIDs; second, for continued uncontrolled pain of a mild to moderate nature, the addition of a weak opioid; and third, for continued uncontrolled pain of a moderate to severe nature, the substitution of a stronger opioid. While it provides a useful guideline, the strict application of the WHO approach to chronic noncancer pain is problematic for several reasons: (1) growing concern regarding the significant morbidity and mortality related to long-term NSAID use, (2) controversy regarding the safety and efficacy of opioids in noncancer pain, and (3) the development of new antiepileptic drugs and other agents that may provide safer alternatives to opioids for certain types of chronic pain.

Clinicians must individualize pain management regimens per patient. The goals of therapy are not only to reduce or control pain, but also to improve daily functioning, physical capabilities, sleep function, and mood.[7] These goals will determine the need for and choice of pharmacologic agents.

Nonpharmacologic therapies can enhance pain control and improve daily functioning. Adjunctive therapies to consider include cognitive-behavioral training, occupational therapy, vocational training, physical therapy, and individual or family therapy.[2,9] Availability of these resources is dependent on practice setting. Pain management clinics may provide many of these services in one coordinated setting. They are also often the source of anesthetic or neurosurgical procedures for pain management.

Nonopioid Analgesics

The nonopioid analgesics—acetaminophen and NSAIDs—are frequently used, although not without safety concerns, for almost all types of chronic pain. These drugs are effective alone for mild to moderate pain and have a synergistic effect when used in combination with opioids for severe pain. They are nonaddictive, antipyretic, and, except for acetaminophen, have an antiinflammatory effect. The nonopioid drugs have an analgesic ceiling—dosage increases beyond recommended levels do not produce further analgesia (Table 9.1).

Acetaminophen

Acetaminophen (Tylenol, others) is recommended for noninflammatory osteoarthritis and other causes of mild to moderate pain. It is safe for patients with renal insufficiency, although liver toxicity can occur in cases of overdose or chronic alcoholism. Some chronic pain patients may require maximum doses of 4 g per day for at least 1 week to determine effectiveness.[10]

Nonacetylated Salicylates

Salsalate (Disalcid and others) and choline magnesium trisalicylate (Trilisate and others) produce analgesic levels similar to aspirin but with less gastropathy and less inhibition of platelet function than aspirin.[11] Nonacetylated salicylates have not been shown to reduce the risk of gastropathy compared to other NSAIDs.

NSAIDs

NSAIDs produce superior analgesia compared with aspirin when given in recommended doses.[11] However, their analgesic effectiveness varies per patient so that several drugs may need to be tried before some patients will report a response. NSAIDs have multiple adverse effects as listed in Table 9.1.[6] Gastrointestinal toxicity is the most frequently reported adverse effect[12] and can lead to significant morbidity and mortality.

Risk factors for NSAID-related gastropathy are (1) age older than 65 years, (2) previous history of peptic ulcer disease (PUD), (3) high doses or multiple types of NSAIDs, (4) concomitant glucocorticoid use, and (5) duration of treatment less than 3 months. The greatest risk of NSAID-related PUD occurs within the first month of therapy.[6]

Recommended methods to reduce the risk of gastropathy are the following[6,12]: (1) Use alternative drugs, if possible. (2) Use the lowest effective dose possible and discontinue, if possible. (3) For patients with two or more risk factors, use concomitant misoprostol (Cytotec), a synthetic prostaglandin analogue that has been shown to decrease gastrointestinal complications of NSAID use by 40%. The recommended dose of misoprostol is 200 μg four times daily but lower doses of 200 μg twice daily may be effective and may help to limit side effects of abdominal cramping and diarrhea. (4) Histamine-2 blockers, e.g., ranitidine (Zantac) or famotidine (Pepcid), have been shown to reduce the incidence of gastric and duodenal ulcers when given prophylactically to patients on chronic NSAID therapy, but the studies are not definitive. (5) Proton pump inhibitors, e.g., omeprazole (Prilosec), also may be effective as preventive agents for NSAID-related gastropathy but add significant cost. (6) Selective COX-2 inhibitor NSAIDs, e.g., celecoxib (Celebrex) and rofecoxib (Vioxx), cause fewer gastrointestinal complications than nonselective agents. They also do not inhibit platelet aggregation and can be used for patients on warfarin. They can cause all of the other adverse effects associated with NSAIDs. They are not more effective analgesics than nonselective NSAIDs.

Table 9.1. Selected Nonopioid Analgesics[6,9–12]

Drug name	Usual dose	Maximum dose	Comments
Acetaminophen (Tylenol, others)	500–1000 mg po q4–6h	4000 mg/d	Recommended for noninflammatory osteoarthritis. May require maximum dose for 1 week for chronic pain trial. Avoid with chronic alcoholism.
Salsalate (Disalcid others)	1000 mg po q8–12h	3000 mg/d	Nonacetylated salicylates produce similar analgesia to, but less gastropathy than aspirin. Minimal antiplatelet activity.
Ibuprofen (Motrin, others)	400–800 mg po q4–6h	3200 mg/d	NSAIDs in recommended doses usually provide superior analgesia compared with aspirin, but do not produce the same analgesic effect in all patients. Major adverse effects are:
Naproxen (Naprosyn, others)	500 mg po q12h	1250 mg/d	1. Elevated blood pressure especially in the elderly and in conjunction with beta-blockers or angiotensin-converting enzyme inhibitors
Indomethacin (Indocin)	25–50 mg po q8h or SR-75 mg po q12h	200 mg/d	2. Fluid retention in patients with congestive heart failure
Ketorolac (Toradol, others)	Pts <65 years: 30 mg IM/IV q6h	120 mg/d	3. Acute renal failure or renal insufficiency 4. Drowsiness and confusion 5. Reversible inhibition of platelet aggregation
	Pts ≥65 years: 15 mg IM/IV q6h	60 mg/d 60 mg/d	6. Anaphylaxis in aspirin-sensitive patients 7. Peptic ulcer disease, regardless of mode (continued)

Table 9.1 (Continued).

Drug name	Usual dose	Maximum dose	Comments
Diclofenac (Cataflam, Voltaren)	50 mg po q8h or SR-75 mg po q12h	150 mg/d	of administration, especially in the first month of therapy.
Nabumetone (Relafen)	1000–1500 mg po qd	1500 mg/d	
Celecoxib (Celebrex)	100–200 mg po q12h	400 mg/d	Selective COX-2 inhibitors and NSAIDs have demonstrated decreased gastrointestinal complications compared with nonselective NSAIDs. They do not inhibit platelet aggregation.
Rofecoxib (Vioxx)	25–50 mg po q24h	50 mg/d	

COX = cyclooxygenase; NSAID = nonsteroidal antiinflammatory drug; SR = sustained release.

Sucralfate (Carafate) and buffered aspirin provide no benefit in the prevention of NSAID-related gastropathy. While enteric-coating of aspirin or naproxen would seem to reduce the risk of topical gastric damage by transferring absorption to the small intestine, there are insufficient data to suggest an overall reduction in gastrointestinal complications.

Opioid Analgesics

The use of opioid analgesics for chronic noncancer pain remains controversial. A recent survey of primary care physicians indicated that, while most physicians are willing to prescribe low potency opioids on an as-needed basis for chronic noncancer pain, a significant portion are unwilling to use higher potency opioids on an around-the-clock basis.[13]

Rationale

The rationale for the use of opioids to alleviate chronic pain is based on the recognition that some patients do not respond to or cannot tolerate other therapy. Physicians' concerns about chronic use of opioids center around three clinical issues: (1) efficacy, (2) safety, and (3) risk of addiction. Available studies of opioid use in noncancer patients suggest the following conclusions regarding these concerns[3,5,14]: (1) Efficacy. Opioids are effective for many types of chronic noncancer pain. Unlike nonopioids, there is no ceiling analgesic effect so that opioids can be titrated up to achieve adequate analgesia. Unfortunately, studies do not demonstrate that this improved analgesic effect is associated with improved daily functioning. (2) Safety: Gastrointestinal and CNS side effects are usually not a problem with long-term opioid use because of the rapid development of tolerance to most of these side effects including nausea, vomiting, cognitive impairment, respiratory depression, and sedation. Constipation can usually be managed with prophylactic use of stool softeners and fiber laxatives. Unlike NSAIDs, there is no known direct organ damage associated with long-term opioid use. (3) Risk of addiction: The risk of inducing opioid addiction among patients with legitimate chronic pain is minimal, although not absent. Long-term opioid therapy often induces *physical dependence*, which is the occurrence of withdrawal symptoms after cessation, and may induce *tolerance*, which is the need for increasing doses to achieve the same analgesic effect. Neither of these physiologic phenomena cause *ad-*

diction, which is a pattern of compulsive behaviors centered around the desire for, acquisition of, and use of the drug. Additional caution and more extensive evaluation are warranted before using chronic opioids for patients with a history of chemical dependency.

There are also legal and regulatory disincentives to prescribing chronic opioid therapy,[3,5,14,15] including diversion of drugs for non-medical uses, diversion of drugs for treatment of narcotics withdrawal, and physicians' fears of licensing or regulatory scrutiny and sanctions for prescribing controlled substances.

Indications/Contraindications

Opioids should be considered for patients with chronic pain who are refractory to other treatments and who have shown responsiveness to opioids.[5] Relative contraindications to starting chronic opioid therapy are a history of substance abuse, drug-seeking behaviors, personality disorders, hepatic insufficiency, renal insufficiency, severe respiratory disease with impaired respiratory drive, preexisting constipation or urinary retention, suicidal tendency, or cognitive impairment.[16]

Guidelines for Therapy

Patients should be educated regarding the goals of therapy; the potential for side effects; the meaning and risks of developing physical dependence, tolerance, and addiction; and the method and schedule for monitoring their use of the drug. A "one physician–one pharmacy" policy should be considered. A patient contract documenting the patient's understanding of these issues should be kept in the medical record.[3,5,15]

Specific Opioids

Table 9.2 lists the commonly used opioid analgesics. Tramadol (Ultram) is an opioid agonist that also blocks norepinephrine and serotonin reuptake. Its effectiveness and side effects are similar to those of weak opioids and may be minimized by gradual titration up to the recommended dose.[10] Physical dependence has been reported but abuse potential is low; therefore, tramadol is not scheduled as a controlled substance.[17] Tramadol may increase the risk of seizures among patients who are at risk for seizures or who are also taking selective serotonin reuptake inhibitors (SSRIs), tricyclic antidepressants (TCAs), opioids, monoamine oxidase inhibitors (MAOIs), or neuroleptics.[4,10]

Meperidine (Demerol) is poorly absorbed orally and cannot be used for patients with impaired renal function or those taking MAOIs be-

Table 9.2. Selected Opioid Analgesics[8,11]

Drug name	Usual dose	Equianalgesic dose to 10 mg oral morphine	Comments
Tramadol (Ultram)	50 mg po tid-qid	—	Slow titration to effective dose may limit side effects.
Codeine (Tylenol #2, #3, #4, others)	30–60 mg po q3–4h	70 mg po	Available in combination with nonopioids, as single agent, as an elixir and injectable.
Hydrocodone (Vicodin, Lortab)	5–10 mg po q3–4h	10 mg po	Only available in combination with nonopioids.
Oxycodone (Percocet, others)	5–10 mg po q3–4h	5–10 mg po	Usually in combination with nonopioids, also as an elixir and as 12-hour sustained-release OxyContin.
Morphine	20–60 mg po q3–4h Sustained-release (MS Contin) 15–60 mg po q12h 10 mg IM/IV q3–6h	— — 3 mg IM/IV	Also available as rectal suppository.
Fentanyl (Duragesic)	25–100 µg/h patch q72h	—	Maximum dose of transdermal patch is 300 µg/hr.

cause of the risk of seizures and other CNS toxicity.[16] The agonist-antagonist group of opioids—pentazocine (Talwin), butorphanol (Stadol), nalbuphine (Nubain), and buprenorphine (Buprenex)—have moderate to strong analgesic potential, but unlike morphine and the other pure agonist drugs, they exhibit an analgesic ceiling. They offer no advantage in analgesic effect or avoidance of side effects. If given to a patient already on a pure agonist drug such as morphine, they precipitate withdrawal symptoms.[5]

Propoxyphene (Darvon, Darvocet) is a nonopiate narcotic that binds to opioid receptors but is no more effective than acetaminophen and causes significant side effects including nausea, vomiting, constipation, dizziness, cardiac toxicity, and chemical dependency.[10]

Fentanyl is the only opioid available transdermally (Duragesic). It is also available as an oral lozenge (Actiq) for acute pain and in parenteral form (Sublimaze). Because of its slow onset of action, the fentanyl patch is appropriate for patients already on opioids who have constant pain with few pain breakthrough episodes. Individual dosing varies greatly owing to differences in skin absorption.[16]

Dosing

Patients with only episodic pain do well with intermittent dosing of opioids. Those with more frequent or continuous symptoms should be given doses around the clock, with rescue doses for sudden exacerbations of pain. Patients with relatively steady pain who are on longer-acting opioids also require occasional rescue doses in the form of shorter-acting agents. Patients in whom sedation may be particularly hazardous because of their occupations can be started at lower than recommended doses of opioids and be titrated upward to build tolerance to the sedative effects. Patients who develop persistent side effects to one opioid may do better with another. The dosages of some products are limited by being placed in combination with acetaminophen or aspirin.[5,16]

Discontinuation

Discontinuation of opioids should be considered in the event that the underlying cause of the pain is resolved, other pain management strategies are providing sufficient pain relief, if unacceptable side effects develop, or if abuse behavior occurs. Discontinuation of chronic opioid therapy can be achieved without precipitating withdrawal symptoms by gradually tapering the dose over 1 to 4 weeks. Clonidine (oral dose 0.05–0.2 mg every 6 hours) can be used to inhibit withdrawal symptoms during opioid tapering. Dosing should be adjusted based on the patient's blood pressure and level of sedation induced by clonidine. Benzodiazepines may also be used to reduce irritability and anxiety during opioid withdrawal.[5,15]

Adjuvant Agents

Antidepressants

Although their mechanism is unknown, TCAs are effective in the treatment of neuropathic pain such as diabetic neuropathy or postherpetic neuralgia.[9,14] Amitriptyline (Elavil) is commonly used in low initial doses of 10 to 25 mg at bedtime with gradual upward titration as needed and as tolerated. There are less data supporting the use of SSRIs for chronic neuropathic pain, but SSRIs do not produce the anticholinergic side effects and cardiac conduction abnormalities associated with TCAs and are effective in treating the depression, insomnia, and anxiety associated with chronic pain.

Antiepileptics

Traditional antiepileptic drugs (AEDs) such as carbamazepine (Tegretol), phenytoin (Dilantin), and valproate (Depakote) are effective for many types of neuropathic pain, but their use may be limited by side effects and drug interactions. Of the newer AEDs, initial research shows gabapentin (Neurontin) is a safe, effective drug for neuropathic pain with few drug interactions.[4,9,14] Its onset of analgesic effect may be more rapid than TCAs and it may be opioid sparing. Its mechanism of action is unknown. Dosing begins at 100 to 300 mg daily, increasing to 900 mg daily in 3 days with an additional increase of 100 to 300 mg every week until therapeutic effect is achieved. Most reports suggest dosages for chronic neuropathic pain are 1800 to 3600 mg daily in three to four divided doses.

Baclofen

Baclofen (Lioresal) is a GABA analogue that, by binding to GABA receptors in the spinal cord, alters CNS control of pain.[14] It is used for neuropathic pain, particularly trigeminal neuralgia. The usual daily dose is 20 to 60 mg divided into three to four doses. Side effects are sedation, weakness, dizziness, nausea, and confusion.

Capsaicin

Capsaicin (Zostrix Cream), derived from jalapeno peppers, is a topical agent useful for osteoarthritis localized to a few joints.[10] Its mechanism of action is depletion of substance P in peripheral nociceptors. It is available over the counter, may be applied two to four times daily, and has no serious side effects. Application site burning or stinging reduces with continued use.

References

1. Newberger PE, Sallan SE. Chronic pain: principles of management. J Pediatr 1981;98(2):180–9.
2. Russo CM, Brosse WG. Chronic pain. Annu Rev Med 1998;49:123–33.
3. Barnsworth B. Risk-benefit assessment of opioids in chronic noncancer pain. Drug Safety 1999;21(4):283–96.
4. Hanson HC. Treatment of chronic pain with antiepileptic drugs: a new era. South Med J 1999;92(7):642–9.
5. Savage SR. Opioid use in the management of chronic pain. Med Clin North Am 1999;83(3):761–86.
6. Brooks P. Use and benefits of nonsteroidal anti-inflammatory drugs. Am J Med 1998;104(3A):9S–13S.
7. World Health Organization. Cancer pain relief and palliative care: report of a WHO expert committee. Geneva, Switzerland: World Health Organization, 1990.
8. Montauk SL. Treating chronic pain. Am Fam Physician 1997;55(4):1151–60.
9. Marcus D. Treatment of nonmalignant chronic pain. Am Fam Physician 2000;61(5):1331–8.
10. Schnitzer TJ. Non-NSAID pharmacologic treatment options for the management of chronic pain. Am J Med 1998;105(1B):45S–52S.
11. Drugs for pain. Med Lett 2000;42(1085):73–8.
12. Ament PW, Childers RS. Prophylaxis and treatment of NSAID-induced gastropathy. Am Fam Physician 1997;55(4):1323–32.
13. Potter M, Schafer S, et al. Opioids for chronic nonmalignant pain. J Fam Pract 2001;50(2):145–51.
14. Pappagallo M. Aggressive pharmacologic treatment of pain. Rheum Dis Clin North Am 1999;25(1):193–213.
15. Longo LP, Parran T. Addiction: part II. Identification and management of the drug-seeking patient. Am Fam Physician 2000;61(8):2401–8.
16. Brown RL, Fleming M. Chronic opioid analgesic therapy for chronic low back pain. J Am Board Fam Pract 1996;9(3):191–204.
17. Cicero TJ, Adams EH. A postmarketing surveillance program to monitor Ultram abuse in the United States. Drug Alcohol Depend 1999;57(1):7–22.

10

Care of the
Dying Patient

Frank S. Celestino

Family physicians have traditionally prided themselves on comprehensive and continuous provision of care throughout the human life cycle. When managing the terminal phases of illness, however, most clinicians have had little formal education directed at the experience of human suffering and dying.[1,2] For many physicians the task and challenge of caring for a dying patient can seem overwhelming. The aging of the United States population, the development and widespread use of life-prolonging technologies, the ascendence of managed care emphasizing the central role of the primary care physician, media attention, the growing discomfort with futile treatment, the public's interest in physician-assisted suicide and the demand for better palliation have all fueled a growing need for physicians to master the art and science of helping patients achieve death with dignity.[3–5] This need has led to a series of major initiatives to improve palliative care education for both clinicians and the public, including the Education for Physicians in End-of-Life Care Project of the American Medical Association, the Faculty Scholars in End-of-Life Care Program of the Department of Veteran Affairs, the Improving Residency Training in End-of-Life Care Program of the American Board of Internal Medicine, the Project on Death in America of the Soros Foundation, and the Last Acts Program of the Robert Wood Johnson Foundation.[3,6]

This chapter reviews the key components of a comprehensive care program for terminally ill patients (Table 10.1).[7–9] The focus is on

Table 10.1. **Components of a Comprehensive Care Plan for Dying Patients**

Compassionate and professional communication of diagnosis, treatment options, and prognosis

Psychosocial support of the patient and family

    Includes developing an understanding of the cultural and religious (spiritual) meaning of suffering and death for the patient and family

    Emphasizes continuity to allay fears of abandonment

Implementation of a comprehensive, evidence-based palliative care program

    Multidisciplinary in nature (physicians, nurses, clergy, social workers, pharmacists, nutritionists, lawyers, patient advocates)

    Hospice involvement

    Establishment and clarification of advance care directives (living wills, durable power of attorney for health care, autopsy and organ donation wishes, dying in hospital versus at home), and attitudes toward physician-assisted suicide

    Pain management (WHO and ACS guidelines)

    Nonpain symptom treatment (including behavioral/psychiatric issues)

    Nutritional support

Acknowledgment and management of financial and reimbursement issues

Bereavement management

WHO = World Health Organization; ACS = American Cancer Society.

optimum care of patients who experience prolonged but predictable dying. Classically, these individuals have had disseminated cancer. It is now recognized that a much broader array of dying patients—those with acquired immunodeficiency syndrome, end-stage renal or cardiac disease, emphysema, and degenerative neurologic diseases—deserve such comprehensive palliative care. For a more detailed discussion of the topics covered in this chapter, the reader can consult two recent theme issues that exhaustively review the cultural, spiritual, political, ethical, economic, social, and medical aspects of terminal care.[10,11]

Cultural Context of Dying and Suffering

The last 50 years have witnessed the increasing medicalization of death in the United States, with most patients now dying in hospitals instead of at home.[3,9–12] The Council on Scientific Affairs of the

American Medical Association (AMA)[9] has emphasized that "in the current system of care, many dying patients suffer needlessly, burden their families, and die isolated from families and community." The AMA council and others[3,6] have cited the advance directives movement, the rising public enthusiasm for euthanasia and physician-assisted suicide, the popularity of the hospice, sensationalized court cases, and the establishment of organizations such as Americans for Better Care of the Dying and the Hemlock Society as evidence of increasing uneasiness with medicine's response to dying. They call for acceptance of dying as a normal part of the human life cycle, expanded research into terminal care, educational programs for all health professionals, and better reimbursement for terminal care.[5,6]

Communication of Diagnosis, Therapy Plans, and Prognosis

Several recent reviews have highlighted a number of sources of communication difficulties with dying patients, including social factors, patient and family barriers, and issues specific to physicians.[13–17] Buckman[13] addressed two specific tasks of communication in terminal care: breaking bad news and engaging in therapeutic dialogue. His six-step protocol is a useful paradigm for all health care practitioners: (1) getting started, which includes such issues as location, eye contact, personal touch, timing, and participants; (2) finding out how much the patient already knows and understands; (3) learning how much the patient wants to know; (4) sharing appropriate amounts of information, with attention to aligning and educating; (5) responding to the patient's and family's feelings; and (6) planning ongoing care and follow-through.

There is usually no reason to provide detailed answers to questions the patient has not yet asked. The concept of gradualism—revealing the total truth in small doses as the illness unfolds—allows the patient the opportunity to develop appropriate coping strategies. However, it is important not to use euphemisms (such as swelling or lump), but to acknowledge the presence of cancer when confirmation is in hand. One must also realize that many patients do not hear the bad news accurately when it is first presented, and reexplanation is often needed.

Not only has the primacy of patient autonomy in modern medicine encouraged truth telling, but studies reveal that patients greatly prefer open, honest communication.[13–17] Overall, the drive for disclosure must be counterbalanced by the realization that the terminally ill patient struggles to maintain a sense of hope in the face of an increasingly ominous medical situation. Clinicians must continue to nurture hope in their dying patients through appropriate optimism around aspects of treatment, achievable goals, and prognosis, combined with timely praise for the patient and family's efforts to achieve spiritual healing and death with dignity. When physicians apply good communication skills (including attending to both verbal and nonverbal signals, exploring incongruent affect, and empathically eliciting patients' perspectives) and actively work to reduce barriers to mutual understanding, patients experience a reduction in both physical and psychological aspects of suffering.

One of the most difficult tasks is predicting how long the patient will live. With improved computing and statistical tools, more accurate objective estimates of survival are often available.[18] Despite these advances prognostication for many patients remains an imperfect science. One approach is to provide a conservative estimate that allows the patient and family to feel proud about "beating the odds" and exceeding expectations.

Psychosocial Support of the Patient and Family

One of the greatest challenges facing clinicians is to adequately address the multitude of psychosocial needs of dying patients and their families.[19] Kubler-Ross was one of the first to study and popularize the notion that terminally ill individuals often experience predictable stages of emotional adaptation and response to the dying process.[20] The five stages were characterized as shock and denial, anger, bargaining, depression, and acceptance. Although duration of these stages and the intensity and sequencing with which they are experienced are highly variable from one individual to the next, accurate recognition of the patient's psychological stage allows the clinician to optimize communication, support, and empathy to meet new needs as they arise.

In addition to the needs delineated in Table 10.1, and the desire for truth telling and a sense of hopefulness, dying patients above almost all else want assurance that the physician (and others) will not abandon them.[21] There is often great fear of dying alone in an environment separated from loved ones and worry about being repulsive to others because of loss of control over bodily functions. Terminally ill patients often seek physical expressions of caring, such as touching, hugging, and kissing. Regardless of their formal involvement with organized religion, they also often seek closure on the spiritual issues of their lives. Many individuals find great solace in life review: the pleasures, pains, accomplishments, and regrets. Most desire some input into making decisions about their care. The above list of concerns applies as much to the family as to the patient. Although in many circumstances family members are critical to the success of terminal care, one must recognize not only caregiver depression and burnout but also dysfunctional family relationships that impede successful physician management.

An often underappreciated aspect of successful supportive care is developing understanding of the symbolic meaning of suffering and dying for the individual patient. Experiences of illness and death and beliefs about the appropriate role of healers are profoundly influenced by a patient's cultural[22] and religious[19,22,23] background. Efforts to use racial or ethnic background alone as predictors of beliefs or behaviors may lead to stereotyping of patients and culturally insensitive care for the dying. Koenig and Gates-Williams[24] provide a protocol to assess the impact of culture. They recommend assessing, in addition to ethnicity, (1) the vocabulary most appropriate for discussing the illness and death; (2) who has decision-making power—the patient or the larger family unit; (3) the relevance of religious beliefs (death, afterlife, miracles, sin); (4) the attitude toward dead bodies; (5) issues of age, gender, and power relationships within both the family and the health care team; and (6) the patient's political and historical context (e.g., poverty, immigrant status, past discrimination) (also see Chapter 1).

Comprehensive Palliative Care

At some point in the course of a chronic illness, it becomes clear that further therapeutic efforts directed at cure or stabilization are futile. Emphasis then shifts from curative to palliative care with an enhanced focus on optimal function and quality of life. According to the World Health Organization (WHO), palliative care "affirms life, regards dying as a normal process, neither hastens nor postpones death, provides relief from pain and other distressing symptoms, integrates the psychological and spiritual aspects of care, offers a support system to help patients live as actively as possible until death and provides support to help the family cope during the patient's illness and in their own bereavement."[25]

Hospice

In the United States, palliative care is most effectively provided by the now more than 2000 hospice organizations that coordinate the provision of high-quality interdisciplinary care to patients and families much more effectively and efficiently than most physicians could do on their own.[26] The first hospice was opened in South London by Dr. Cicely Saunders in 1967, with the concept first appearing in America by 1974. Philosophically, the objectives of hospice and palliative care are the same. Hospice care, which is provided regardless of ability to pay, has grown from an alternative health care movement to an accepted part of the American health care system, with Medicare reimbursement beginning in 1982. Hospice organizations provide a highly qualified, specially trained interdisciplinary team of professionals (nurses, pharmacists, counselors, pastoral care, patient care coordinators, volunteers) who work together to meet the physiologic, psychological, social, spiritual, and economic needs of patients and families facing terminal illness.[26] Classically, more than 80% of hospice patients have had disseminated cancer, but in recent years patients with chronic diseases that are deemed inevitably terminal within 6 months have become eligible as well. The hospice team collaborates continuously with the patient's attending physician (who must certify the terminal condition), to develop and maintain a patient-centered, individualized plan of care. Hospice medical services and consultation are available 24 hours a day, 7 days a week, though minute-to-minute personal care of the patient by the hospice team is not feasible and must be provided by family or volunteers. Hospice care, though aimed at allowing the patient to remain at home if desired, continues uninterrupted should the patient need acute hospital care or a hospice inpatient unit.

Advance Directives

Because it is now possible to keep sick patients alive longer at greater cost with lesser quality of life, patients and physicians have welcomed the emphasis on advance directives planning. *Advance directive* is an "umbrella" term that refers to any directive for health care made in advance of serious, cognition-impairing illness that robs the patient of decision-making capability.

Two general types of directive are widely recognized.[27] With the instructional type the patient specifies in writing certain circumstances and, in advance, declines or accepts specific treatments. The second type involves appointment of a health care agent, a person to whom is delegated all authority about medical decisions. Each type of directive has its strengths and drawbacks, and they should be seen as complementary, not competitive.

The advance directives movement seems to fit well with an emphasis on patient autonomy and the economic reality of needing to conserve health costs. Unfortunately, studies have revealed that advance directives may make little difference in the way patients are treated at the end of life and reduce costs only modestly.[28,29] Similar drawbacks have applied to the Patient Self-Determination Act, which when implemented in 1991 was designed to encourage competent adults to complete advance directives and to help identify those patients who previously had executed such documents on admission to acute or long-term facilities. Nonetheless, in practice the discussions among physician, patient, and family leading up to establishment of a formal directive are often of greater importance than the documents themselves. When a terminally ill patient calmly discusses foreseeable events and choices leading up to death, the effect on anxious family members can be dramatic and salutary. Such discussions ideally occur relatively early after a terminal illness is diagnosed so as to avoid a crisis situation in which the patient becomes incapacitated and the family must assume responsibility for clinical decisions in the absence of knowledge about their loved one's preferences. State statutes vary widely regarding living wills and health care proxies as well as the authority granted to close friends or family members in the common situation where an incapacitated person has left no advance directives.

Physicians must realize that most dying patients at some point contemplate suicide and that a small but significant number, in one way or another, will ask their physicians to help hasten death.[30,31] With the publicity surrounding doctor-aided suicides in Michigan and the onslaught of state and federal judicial and legislative activity concerning physician-assisted suicide (PAS), clinicians caring for dying patients must explore their own moral stance in this challenging area so as to deal more effectively with patient suffering. Fortunately, approval of PAS in Oregon (and the Netherlands) has greatly stimulated clinicians' interest in palliative care, especially when abuses of the PAS process are uncovered.[31]

Inherent in any discussion of advance directives is the concept of the loss of "decision-making capacity." This catch-phrase obscures the fact that in common practice decisional capacity is difficult to assess. The elements of capacity seem straightforward: Can the person indicate a choice and do so free of coercion? Can the person manipulate relevant information meaningfully and understand the consequences of choosing each of the options? Searight[32] published a helpful, clinically relevant interview framework for assessing patient medical decision-making capacity. Such approaches verify that early dementia does not by itself usually prevent patients from participating in advance directives discussions.

Pain Management

Symptom management, especially achieving pain relief (see Chapter 9), remains the first priority for the attending physician and palliative care team.[3,7–9,25,33–35] Without effective control of pain and other sources of physical distress, quality of life for the dying patient is unacceptable, and progress on the psychological work of dying is aborted. The very prospect of pain induces fear in the patient, and frustration, anxiety, fatigue, insomnia, boredom, and anger contribute to a lowered threshold for pain. Thus treatment of the entire patient contributes to pain control.

Despite decades of evidence that physicians can and should be successful in controlling cancer pain, studies continue to reveal undertreatment and multiple barriers to effective cancer pain management.[6,33–35] Physicians have been guilty of inadequate knowledge of pain therapies, poor pain assessment, overconcern about controlled substances' regulations, and fear of patient addiction and tolerance. On the other hand, patients may be reluctant to report pain accurately. The health care system also presents impediments by giving cancer pain treatment low priority and inadequate reimbursement, along with restrictive regulation of controlled substances.

Pain during terminal illness and with cancer may be of two types: (1) nociceptive (somatic/visceral) and (2) neuropathic.[25,33–35] Somatic/visceral pain arises from direct stimulation of afferent nerves due to tumor infiltration of skin, soft tissue, or viscera. Somatic pain is often described as dull or aching and is well localized. Bone and soft tissue metastases are examples of somatic pain. Visceral pain tends to be poorly localized and is often referred to dermatomal sites distant from the source of the pain.

Neuropathic pain results from injury to some element of the nervous system because of the direct effect of the tumor or as a result of cancer therapy (surgery, irradiation, or chemotherapy). Examples include brachial or lumbosacral plexus invasion, spinal nerve root compression, or neuropathic complications of drugs such as vincristine. Neuropathic pain is described as sharp, shooting, shock-like, or burning and is often associated with dysesthesias. Unlike somatic/visceral pain, neuropathic pain may be relatively less responsive to opioids, whereas antidepressants, anticonvulsants, or local anesthetics may have good efficacy (also see Chapter 9).

An optimum pain management program includes assessing the pathophysiology of the patient's pain, taking a pain history, noting response to prior therapies, discussing the patient's goals for pain control, assessing psychosocial contributors to pain, and frequently reevaluating the patient after changes in treatment. Use of visual analogue or other pain scales is particularly useful for initial assessment and follow-up. This technique is in keeping with the new Joint Commission on Accreditation of Healthcare Organizations (JCAHO) standards of pain assessment, which encourage viewing pain as a vital sign.

Classically, the management of pain in terminally ill patients has involved multiple modalities: analgesic drugs, psychosocial and emotional support, palliative irradiation and surgery, and anesthesia-related techniques, such as nerve blocks, which can be both diagnostic and therapeutic.[33–35] Sometimes chemotherapy, radiopharmaceuticals, or hormonal therapies are of some help with cancer pain.

Analgesics are the mainstay for management of cancer and terminal illness pain. Traditionally, they have been classified into three broad categories: nonopioids (aspirin, acetaminophen, nonsteroidal antiinflammatory agents), opioids (with morphine the prototype), and adjuvant analgesics (antidepressants, anticonvulsants, local anesthetics, capsaicin, corticosteroids, and neuroleptics).

Because patients with advanced disease often have mixed types of pain, drugs from different classes are often combined to achieve optimal pain relief. This concept, together with the principle of using the simplest dosing schedule and the least-invasive modalities first, form the basis for WHO's "analgesic ladder" approach to pain management.[25] This approach, which has been validated in clinical trials worldwide and championed by other agencies,[25] recommends nonopioids for mild to moderate pain (step 1), adding opioids (including tramadol) for persistent or increasing pain (step 2), and finally increasing the opioid potency or dose as the pain escalates (step 3). At each step, adjuvant medications are considered based on the underlying causes of the pain. The ladder-based protocol should not be seen as rigid, as therapy must always be individualized, with doses and intervals carefully adjusted to provide optimal relief of pain with minimal side effects.

Although many opioid analgesics exist, morphine remains the gold standard. Morphine has a simple metabolic route with no accumulation of clinically significant active metabolites. There are a wide variety of preparations, making it easy to titrate or change routes of administration. When switching narcotics or routes of administration, physicians must be familiar with the well-publicized charts of equianalgesic dosing equivalents.[33–35]

Regardless of the choice of specific drug, doses should be given on a regular schedule, by the clock, to maintain steady blood levels. Additional rescue doses can be superimposed as needed on the baseline regimen. Transdermal fentanyl has been another option for achieving steady-state blood levels.

There is no ceiling effect for morphine dosing. The hallmark of tolerance development is shortening of the duration of analgesic action. Physical dependence is expected, and addiction is rare. Sharp increases in dosage requirements usually imply worsening of the underlying disease. Opioid side effects—constipation, nausea, vomiting, mental clouding, sedation, respiratory depression—are watched for vigilantly, anticipated, and prevented if possible. Constipation is so pervasive an issue that all patients on opioids should be started on a bowel management regimen that may include fluid, fiber, stool softeners, laxatives, enemas, or lactulose.

Regarding adjuvants, corticosteroids provide a range of effects, including mood elevation, antiinflammatory activ-ity, antiemetic effects, appetite stimulation (helpful with cachexia), and reduction of cerebral and spinal cord edema. They may be helpful for bone and nerve pain. Megestrol may also stimulate appetite. Antidepressants in lower doses (e.g., 10–100 mg of the prototype amitriptyline) and anticonvulsants (especially gabapentin) help alleviate neuropathic pain and provide innate analgesia as well as potentiation of opioids. In standard doses the antidepressants are mood elevating, with particularly promising results achieved with the newer selective serotonin reuptake inhibitors. Psychostimulants (e.g., methylphenidate) may be useful for reducing opioid-induced respiratory depression and sedation when dosage adjustment is not feasible. Bisphosphonates and radiopharmaceuticals can be helpful with bone pain.

Physical and psychosocial modalities can be used with drugs to manage pain during all phases of treatment. Physical modalities include cutaneous stimulation, heat, cold, massage, pressure, gentle exercise, repositioning, biofeedback, transcutaneous electrical nerve stimulation, aroma therapy, acupuncture, and even immobilization (casting). A variety of cognitive-behavioral interventions can also be employed: relaxation, guided imagery, distraction, reframing, psychotherapy, and support groups.

Nonpain Symptom Management

Dying patients struggle with numerous losses and fears that are exacerbated by debilitating and often demeaning nonpain symptoms, including nausea, vomiting, anorexia, diarrhea, bowel impaction, depression, anxiety, delirium, cough, dyspnea, visceral or bladder spasms, hiccups, decubiti, and xerostomia. To preclude unnecessary suffering, clinicians must utilize diverse methods to optimize palliative care and provide a relatively symptom-free death.[3,7–9,36] Morphine is of particular help with dyspnea.[33] The key is to search for reversible causes of these diverse symptom complexes before resorting to medication management, which in extreme cases of unrelieved suffering can include legally and morally sanctioned "terminal" sedation (the so-called double-effect phenomenon).[7–9,36]

Anorexia with decreased intake is distressing to families. In addition, concerns about providing adequate nutrition and hydration have arisen on both a moral and symptom relief basis. Studies have revealed that hunger is a rare symptom, and that thirst and dry mouth are usually easily managed with local mouth care and sips.[10,11,37] Thus food and fluid administration are now thought not to play a significant role in providing comfort to terminally ill patients, nor is such provision thought to be morally mandated (though the symbolic meaning of feeding efforts should not be overlooked). Interestingly, force feeding and total parenteral nutrition tend to shorten survival, and tube feedings do not decrease aspiration risk.[37]

Bereavement and Grief

Most family members suffer psychologically during the dying of a loved one and then go through an expected process of bereavement. A multitude of feelings—shock, disbelief, a general numbing of all affect, protest, relief, guilt, anguish, emotional lability, tearfulness—accompany the first days to weeks of grieving, eventually giving way to less intense feelings that in normal circumstances are largely resolved within 1 year. The mourning period is a time of physical vulnerability, with bereaved persons likely to suffer impaired immune status and behavioral problems.[38]

The family physician is often best situated to provide ongoing bereavement services. The 13-month bereavement support offered by hospice agencies and community grief support groups can be utilized. Key tasks for the physician providing care to the bereaved include validating and normalizing feelings, not medicating emotions simply because they are intense, assessing the progress of the family's grief work, identifying and intervening in abnormal grief, and using age-appropriate models and interactional styles.[38] Short-acting benzodiazepines can be helpful during the first 1 to 2 weeks if family members need relief from sleeplessness and extreme tearfulness.

Special Needs of Dying Children

Although most of the previously mentioned principles of comprehensive terminal care apply equally well to dying children, several additional considerations should be emphasized.[39,40] Communication must include age and developmentally appropriate vocabulary. Although most children do not develop an accurate understanding of dying until age 7 to 8, those as young as 4 to 5 recognize that they are gravely ill. Physicians should openly discuss with parents what role they wish to play in discussions of diagnosis, prognosis, and death.

Multidisciplinary hospice involvement may be even more important for children than adults. Likewise, studies have verified that most terminally ill children, as well as their families, fare better when the caring and dying occur at home.[39,40] Clinicians must remain cognizant of sibling issues such as feelings of neglect or jealousy. Siblings may need reassurance that they are not in some way responsible for the child's dying. In general, siblings should be encouraged to participate in the care of their dying loved one.

Conclusion

The challenge in providing terminal care is to form an accurate understanding of the needs and preferences of the dying patient and to fit the delivery of care to those needs. The fundamental rule is that good care involves giving patients options and some sense of control. Physicians must realize that patients' needs are shaped in unusual ways by factors (cultural and religious) that fall outside the comfortable biomedical domain.

References

1. Billings JA, Block S. Palliative care in undergraduate medical education. JAMA 1997;278:733–8.
2. Rabow MW, Hardie GE, Fair JM, McPhee SJ. End-of-life care content in 50 textbooks from multiple specialties. JAMA 2000;283:771–8.

3. Cassell CK, Field MJ, eds. Approaching death: improving care at the end of life. Washington, DC: National Academy Press, 1997.
4. Block SD, Bernier GM, Crawley LM, for the National Consensus Conference on Medical Education for Care Near the End of Life. Incorporating palliative care into primary care education. J Gen Intern Med 1998;13:768–73.
5. Mularski RA. Educational agenda for interdisciplinary end of life curricula. Crit Care Med 2001;29(2 suppl):N16–23.
6. Emmanuel LL, von Gunten CF, Ferris FD. Gaps in end-of-life care. Arch Fam Med 2000;9:1176–80.
7. Task Force on Palliative Care. Precepts of palliative care. J Palliat Med 1998;1:109–12.
8. Cassell CK, Foley KM, eds. Principles for care of patients at the end of life: an emerging consensus among the specialties of medicine. New York: Millbank Memorial Fund, 1999.
9. Council on Scientific Affairs, American Medical Association. Good care of the dying patient. JAMA 1996;275:474–8.
10. Winker MA, Flanagin A, eds. Theme issue: end-of-life care. JAMA 2000;284:2413–528.
11. Matzo ML, Lynn J, eds. Death and dying. Clin Geriatr Med 2000;16:211–398.
12. Fox EJ. Predominance of the curative model of medical care. JAMA 1999;278:761–3.
13. Buckman R. How to break bad news: a guide for health care professionals. Baltimore: Johns Hopkins University Press, 1992.
14. Siegler EL, Levin BW. Physician–older patient communication at the end of life. Clin Geriatr Med 2000;16:175–204.
15. von Gunten CF, Ferris FD, Emanuell LL. Ensuring competency in end of life care—communication and relational skills. JAMA 2000;284:3051–7.
16. Balaban RB. A physician's guide to talking about end of life care. J Gen Intern Med 2000;15:195–200.
17. Quill TE. Initiating end of life discussions with seriously ill patients: addressing the "elephant in the room." JAMA 2000;284:2502–7.
18. Christakis NA. Death foretold: prophecy and prognosis in medical care. Chicago: University of Chicago Press, 2000.
19. Block SD. Psychological considerations, growth, and transcendence at the end of life—the art of the possible. JAMA 2001;285:2898–905.
20. Kubler-Ross E. On death and dying. New York: Macmillan, 1969.
21. Singer PA, Martin DK, Kelner M. Quality end of life care: patient perspectives. JAMA 1999;281:163–8.
22. Vincent JL. Cultural differences in end of life care. Crit Care Med 2001;29(2 suppl):N52–5.
23. Daaleman TP, VandeCreek L. Placing religion and spirituality in end of life care. JAMA 2000;284:2514–7.
24. Koenig BA, Gates-Williams J. Understanding cultural differences in caring for dying patients. West J Med 1995;163:244–9.
25. Jadad AR, Bowman GP. The WHO analgesic ladder for cancer pain management. JAMA 1995;274:1870–3.

26. Lynn J. Serving patients who may die soon—the role of hospice and other services. JAMA 2001;285:925–32.
27. Fischer GS, Arnold RM, Tulsky JA. Talking to the older adult about advance directives. Clin Geriatr Med 2000;16:239–54.
28. Lynn J. Rethinking fundamental assumptions: SUPPORT's implications for future reform. J Am Geriatr Soc 2000;48:S214–21.
29. Emanuel EJ. Cost savings at the end of life: what do the data show? JAMA 1996;275:1907–14.
30. Emanuell LL. Facing requests for physician-assisted suicide—toward a practical and principled clinical skill set. JAMA 1998;280:643–7.
31. Nuland SB. Physician-assisted suicide and euthanasia in practice. N Engl J Med 2000;342:583–4.
32. Searight HR. Assessing patient competence for medical decision making. Am Fam Physician 1992;45:751–9.
33. Cherny NI. The management of cancer pain. CA 2000;50:70–116.
34. Abrahm JL. Advances in pain management for older adult patients. Clin Geriatr Med 2000;16:269–311.
35. Chang HM. Cancer pain management. Med Clin North Am 1999;83: 711–36.
36. Bruera E, Neumann CM. Management of specific symptom complexes in patients receiving palliative care. Can Med Assoc J 1998;158: 1717–26.
37. Huang Z, Ahronheim C. Nutrition and hydration in terminally ill patients: an update. Clin Geriatr Med 2000;16:313–25.
38. Casarett D, Kutner JS, Abrahm J, for the ACP-ASIM End of Life Consensus Panel. Life after death—a practical approach to grief and bereavement. Ann Intern Med 2001;134:208–15.
39. Masri C, Farrell CA, Lacroix J, Rocker G, Shesnie SD. Decision-making and end of life care in critically-ill children. J Palliat Care 2000;16(suppl):S45–52.
40. American Academy of Pediatrics Committee on Bioethics and Committee on Hospital Care. Palliative care for children. Pediatrics 2000; 106:351–7.

11

Diseases of the Rectum and Anus

Thomas J. Zuber

Anorectal disorders represent some of the most common, yet poorly understood conditions in primary care. Any discussion of these conditions requires a thorough understanding of the anorectal anatomy (Figs. 11.1 and 11.2). The anal canal spans 2 to 3 cm from the lower border of the anal crypts at the dentate line to the anal verge (external skin).[1] The anal canal is lined with a specialized squamous epithelium called anoderm.[1] Sensory innervation from the external skin extends upward to the dentate line. Most patients have no sensation above the dentate line and are exquisitely sensitive below it.

Internal and external hemorrhoids are discussed here in detail, as patients often attribute all anorectal complaints to "hemorrhoids." Other conditions that are reviewed include anal fissures, abscesses, fistulas, incontinence, rectal prolapse, pruritus ani, infectious proctitis, hidradenitis suppurativa, condyloma acuminatum, and anal carcinoma.

Hemorrhoids

It is estimated that 50% to 75% of United States adults suffer at some time from hemorrhoids.[2,3] Hemorrhoids are distended vascular cushions that line the anal canal.[4–7] Internal hemorrhoids are composed, in part, of the dilated terminal tributaries of the superior and middle rectal veins, appearing above the dentate line.[2] External hemorrhoids are composed of the dilated tributaries of the inferior rectal vein, ap-

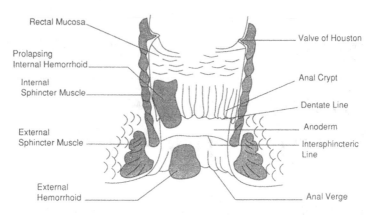

Fig. 11.1. Anorectal anatomy and hemorrhoids.

pearing below the dentate line[2] (Fig. 11.1). Mixed hemorrhoids are composed of both internal and external hemorrhoids.

The anal cushions are composed of arterioles and venules,[6,7] so describing internal hemorrhoids as simple "varicose veins" is inaccurate. The submucosal anchoring and connective tissue structure inside an anal cushion can become worn by chronic straining or from trauma from passing inspissated stool.[3] Ablative treatments for internal hemorrhoids attempt to re-create connective tissue anchoring by scarring the mucosa to the underlying tissues.[3]

The entire anal canal must be thoroughly investigated before initiating treatment for hemorrhoids. Patients can be examined in the knee-chest position, but most practitioners prefer the Sims' or left lateral decubitus position. The slotted Ives anoscope (Redfield Corporation, Montvale, NJ) provides excellent visualization of a full anal cushion or hemorrhoids above and below the dentate line. Once the pathology is identified, patients can be offered appropriate treatment interventions for their stage or severity of disease (Table 11.1).

Hemorrhoids tend to be a recurring problem.[5] Lifestyle changes are important to limit the need for repeated treatments and should be recommended for all patients.[4] The initial use of stool softeners and the long-term use of stool bulking agents can reduce straining and trauma to the anal canal.[4,5,8–10] Patients should be encouraged to drink six full glasses of water a day and consume at least five servings of fresh fruits and fresh vegetables daily.[9] Prolonged sitting should be avoided, and patients should be educated not to delay toileting once the rectum fills.

Table 11.1. **Grading and Treatment Recommendations for Internal Hemorrhoids**

Grade	Appearance	Treatment options
I	Excessive bulging above the mucosal surface without prolapse	Conservative management with fiber, stool bulking agents, dietary vegetables
II	Prolapse with defecation and spontaneous reduction	Dietary management Infrared coagulation Electrosurgical ablation Rubber band ligation
III	Prolapse that requires manual reduction	Infrared coagulation Electrosurgical ablation Rubber band ligation Surgical or laser hemorrhoidectomy
IV	Prolapse that cannot be reduced manually	Surgical hemorrhoidectomy Laser hemorrhoidectomy Electrosurgical ablation

Internal Hemorrhoids

Most patients with internal hemorrhoids present with painless rectal bleeding. Internal hemorrhoids generally develop at the fixed positions of the anal cushions within the anal canal[2,4,5,8] (Fig. 11.2). Several new ablative techniques offer effective, less expensive treatments (Table 11.1). Patients with severe bleeding, persistent prolapse, or failure to respond to conservative modalities may require surgical intervention.[5]

The rubber band ligation technique effectively strangulates the internal hemorrhoid.[1,3] A small rubber band is loaded onto a hollow applicator, the hemorrhoid is pulled inside the applicator, and the rubber band is released to the base of the hemorrhoid.[1,5,8] The hemorrhoid sloughs off during the following 1 to 2 weeks.[3] Moderate pain can follow this procedure, as can the rare but significant complication of pelvic sepsis.[8,11] Any patient with pelvic pain, fever, and inability to urinate following rubber band ligation must be immediately evaluated for this potentially fatal complication.[11]

Infrared photocoagulation is an easily performed office treatment for internal hemorrhoids.[3] A 15-volt tungsten-halogen lamp provides a controlled energy emission at the tip of the instrument.[3] The energy causes tissue destruction up to 3 mm in depth, and subsequent scar formation tethers the hemorrhoidal vessels to the underlying tissues and reduces blood flow into the hemorrhoid.[3] Multiple timed

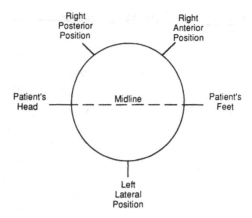

Fig. 11.2. When examining a patient who is lying in the left lateral decubitus (Sims') position, the patient's head is to the left and the feet are to the right. The midline of the canal is parallel to the floor. The circle represents the dentate line. The three anal cushions (and locations for the development of internal hemorrhoids) generally are located at the 10 o'clock position (right posterior), 2 o'clock position (right anterior), and 6 o'clock position (left lateral). This type of circular drawing can be included in the patient's chart when evaluating hemorrhoids, with pathology drawn inside (above the dentate line) or outside the circle to document disease location and severity.

pulses lasting 1.0 to 1.5 seconds are administered at the upper (proximal) portion of the internal hemorrhoid.

Infrared treatments have been described as a "painless" intervention by some authors.[3] Most patients experience a mild burning sensation,[10] but the treatment is performed without anesthesia and is well tolerated. Pelvic sepsis has not been noted following infrared treatment.

Bipolar diathermy and galvanic destruction are two methods of electrosurgical destruction of internal hemorrhoids.[3] Both treatments appear to be effective and safe, and each can be used for higher grade (grade 3 or 4) hemorrhoids. The galvanic destruction technique requires at least 10 minutes of treatment time, compared to a few seconds for infrared or bipolar diathermy treatments.

Some therapies for internal hemorrhoids have been largely discontinued. Sclerotherapy has significant risks, including mucosal sloughing, thrombosis, abscess formation, and bacteremia.[5] Cryotherapy has a high cure rate but produces tremendous watery discharge and can result in sphincter muscle damage and anal stenosis.[3,5] Surgical excision is occasionally required, but other destructive modalities can be employed first. Laser hemorrhoidectomy is expensive and is associated with slower healing rates than standard surgical excision.[12]

External Hemorrhoids

Uncomplicated, nonthrombosed external hemorrhoids rarely require surgical intervention.[5] Novice examiners may mistake external tags for a true external hemorrhoid.[2] A tag results from a prior hemorrhoid that has thrombosed, scarred, and effectively lost its blood supply.[2] Rarely tags cause itching or interfere with hygiene, but they generally are left untreated.

Thrombosed external hemorrhoids can cause extreme pain and disability and are common in pregnant patients and young adults.[13] Patients present with a tender perianal mass, and the bluish blood clot often can be seen through the skin. If the patient presents with the thrombosed hemorrhoid during the first few days or if it ruptures, excision of the thrombosed hemorrhoid is indicated.[5,8] Simple incision and drainage of the clot frequently results in spontaneous reclosure of the skin, rethrombosis, and recurrent pain in 24 hours.[5,8]

Excision of a thrombosed external hemorrhoid can be facilitated by adequate exposure created by an assistant retracting the buttocks laterally.[5] Lidocaine (1–2%) can be administered above and around the hemorrhoid. An elliptical excision is performed, removing overlying skin and the entire clot.[1,5,14] Electrocautery can be employed for hemostasis, and the wound can be left open or closed with a running subcuticular absorbable suture.

Thrombosed hemorrhoids that have been present for more than 48 to 72 hours generally are best treated conservatively.[5,14,15] After 3 days time, the pain produced by surgical intervention frequently is greater than the pain that occurs with spontaneous resolution. The mass usually reduces slowly over the next few weeks.[5]

Nonhemorrhoidal Anorectal Diseases

Anal Fissure

A fissure is a crack or tear in the anal mucosa, usually produced by the passage of hard stool.[16,17] The lesion classically is associated with bleeding and intense pain at defecation.[16,17] Patients often complain of a sharp, cutting, or tearing sensation. Nearly half of the patients present with the complaint of hemorrhoids.[16]

Anal fissures most commonly appear in the midline of the anal canal, with 90% in the posterior midline.[8,16,17] Fissures outside the midline can be associated with other disease states such as Crohn's disease, tuberculosis, or syphilis.[8] A search for associated pathology should be initiated whenever a fissure is found outside the midline.

Because fissures develop in the heavily innervated anoderm, the pain of a fissure often is out of proportion to the lesion's size.[9] They can be diagnosed from the history, digital examination, and anoscopy. When examining for fissures, the sphincter muscle spasm can be overcome by gentle but persistent lateral separation of the edges of the anal orifice using traction of the gloved fingers to the side of the anus.[17]

Once discovered, many fissures heal over a few weeks time with rigorous efforts to soften the stools.[8,16] Stool softeners, increased fluid intake, sitz baths, and stool bulking agents may be helpful.[8,9,16] Lidocaine 2% jelly may assist with pain when applied to the tissues just prior to a bowel movement.

Unhealed fissures can give rise to chronic, intermittent, or continuous symptoms.[16] Recurrent tearing of the anoderm with the passage of each stool can result in a chronic fissure. The anal crypt immediately above the chronic fissure (at the dentate line) can become swollen and edematous, resulting in a hypertrophied anal papilla or polyp.[16,17] Distal to the fissure (at the anal verge) may be a larger sentinel skin tag or sentinel pile.[17] This swelling on the outer edge of the anal canal can serve as a marker for a fissure immediately above.[16,17]

The internal anal sphincter muscle may develop spasm from the presence of the overlying fissure. Over time the fissure may deepen, and the spastic muscle becomes fibrotic and contracted.[17] Conservative measures often fail once the muscle becomes fibrosed. Topical nitroglycerin ointment can reduce sphincter muscle contraction while the fissure is healing.[18–20] Early studies used 0.2% ointment; commercially available products in the United States (2% nitroglycerin ointment) generally should be diluted.[19,20] The ointment sometimes produces headaches and syncope in young patients. Botulinum toxin 20 units injected in two divided doses into the anal sphincter on both sides of the canal appears even more effective.[21,22]

Surgery for anal fissures usually is limited to patients who have persisting fissures unresponsive to conservative measures. Lateral internal sphincterotomy, which releases the contracted muscle, is the most widely recommended intervention.[16,17] This surgery is performed by inserting a thin cataract or no. 11 blade through the perianal skin between the external and internal sphincter muscles. The blade is teased toward a gloved finger in the rectum, dividing the fibrotic internal sphincter. The blade should not cut all the way through to the mucosa.[17] Incontinence occasionally results from the procedure, limiting the use of surgery for fissures.

Anorectal Abscess

An anorectal abscess results from cellulitis or infection of the glands and crypts at the dentate line.[8,17,23] Both aerobic and anaerobic bacteria may be noted within an anorectal abscess.[17] Some reports suggest a higher incidence of the abscesses among men. Anorectal abscesses usually are obvious, producing diffuse swelling, erythema, and pain around the anus. Most abscesses are aggravated by sitting, coughing, sneezing, and defecating.[17] Anterior abscesses in women are occasionally confused with Bartholin's abscesses.

Anorectal abscesses are classified according to their location. A common classification system divides them into perianal, ischiorectal, submucous (or high intermuscular), and pelvirectal.[8,17,23] Perianal abscesses represent half of all anorectal abscesses[8] and appear as ovoid swellings in close proximity to the anus. Fluctuance may be noted on the perianal skin, and spontaneous drainage of a perianal abscess commonly occurs.

Ischiorectal abscesses produce a more diffuse, brawny swelling of the entire perianal region.[17] Digital examination may reveal a bulging in the anal canal. High intermuscular abscesses can be difficult to diagnose. They can produce a chronic aching that is relieved once the abscess bursts and drains pus into the rectum.[17]

Anorectal abscesses should be surgically drained upon discovery.[8,17,23] Perianal abscesses can be drained by a cruciate incision (in the shape of a plus sign) made as close as possible to the anal verge.[8] Direct compression of the tissues expresses the pus, and an iodoform gauze drain can be placed within the abscess cavity for 24 hours or replaced for longer treatment periods. Antibiotics should not be used in place of surgical drainage, and their use after drainage is debated.

Anal Fistula

An anal fistula is a chronic granulating tract connecting two epithelial-lined surfaces.[8,17] Simple fistulas usually have a single external skin opening and a single internal opening in the anal canal or rectal mucosa. More complicated fistulas can have a complex course and multiple external openings. The wall of the tract is lined with a thick, tough layer of fibrous tissue.[17]

Anal fistulas most commonly develop following pyogenic abscesses.[8,17] Small crypt abscesses along the dentate line may serve as a reservoir for repeated infection from enteric bacteria.[17] Three fourths of all fistulas are low anal or low intersphincteric fistulas.[17] Low intersphincteric fistulas extend upward from the skin between the external and internal sphincter muscles and then dive through the internal sphincter to the dentate line.

Anal fistulas are predominantly found in middle-aged men.[17] Patients frequently give the history that they had a prior abscess that burst, producing a chronic intermittent discharge.[17] Anal fistulas generally are painless, but when associated with inflammatory bowel disease patients may complain of additional bowel symptoms. When examining a patient with a fistula, inquiry should be made about changes in bowel habits, passage of mucus and blood, abdominal pain, and weight loss.

The anal skin can exhibit a single or multiple fistular openings. An opening may be situated on the summit of a pink or red nodule of granulation tissue, and palpation of the perianal skin may express pus through the opening. Gentle injection of a dye solution or the use of a probe can identify the course of a fistula tract. Probing in the office setting is discouraged, as it may result in pseudotracts and distortion of the anatomy.[8] Any patient identified with a fistula should be referred for definitive surgical care.[8]

Many surgical and ablative procedures have been devised for fistulas. Most authors recommend opening the fistula tract, with healing accomplished by wound granulation or by performing primary closure.[17] Setons made of silk or rubber bands can be threaded through the fistula and tightened sequentially, producing necrosis of the overlying tissues and externalization of the fibrous tract.[17]

Anal Incontinence

Anal incontinence is loss of control of flatus and feces.[17,24] There are many causes for anal incontinence, some of which appear in Table 11.2. Young patients with incontinence may suffer from congenital anorectal deformities, secondary megacolon from chronic constipation, or trauma to the anal sphincter apparatus.[17,24] Ulcerative colitis can produce anorectal abscesses that destroy the sphincter musculature. Mass lesions such as carcinoma, rectal prolapse, or large hemorrhoids also can produce mechanical interference in canal closure and subsequent incontinence.[17]

Table 11.2. **Some Causes of Anal Incontinence**

Congenital abnormalities (before and after surgery), such as ectopic anus

Neurologic conditions such as tabes dorsalis, spina bifida, cerebral vascular accident, dementia

Birth-related neurologic damage to the pelvic floor musculature resulting from compression injury by the head at delivery

Trauma
    Accidental impalement into the anorectal tissues
    Obstetric tears
    Operative trauma (fistula, hemorrhoids)
    Rectal surgery such as internal sphincterotomy, fistulectomy

Secondary megacolon due to chronic constipation

Rectal prolapse

Large prolapsing third- or fourth-degree hemorrhoids

Ulcerative colitis with perirectal abscesses

Carcinoma of the anal canal

Amebic dysentery

Impaction of feces

Old age and general debility

Rectovaginal fistula

Radiation enteritis

Diarrheal states

Functional fecal incontinence is defined as recurrent uncontrolled passage of fecal material in a person without evidence of neurologic or structural etiologies.[25] The new definition suggests that an individual must be at least 4 years of age, and that the incontinence can be associated with either diarrhea or constipation in an individual with a normal anal sphincter structure.[25] The new definition for functional disease includes the 25% of patients with diarrhea-predominant irritable bowel syndrome who experience incontinence.[25]

Older women are particularly at risk for incontinence due to progressive denervation of the pelvic floor musculature from prior birth-related injury.[24] The aging process can produce decreasing resting sphincter pressures, increased colonic transit time, and decreased sensitivity to rectal distention in both genders. Debilitated elderly patients or those with dementia are particularly prone to incontinence. Efforts should be made to establish a routine of daily stooling, fiber, and stool bulking agents to limit soiling by the elderly.

Incontinence frequently is associated with fecal impaction in the elderly.[17] Fecal impaction occurs when a large, firm, immovable mass of stool develops in the rectum owing to incomplete evacuation of stool.[26] Fecal impaction can be managed by breaking up the mass with a gentle gloved finger or instrument and removing the inspissated stool.[17,26]

Rectal Prolapse

Complete rectal prolapse, or procidentia, is the abnormal descent of all layers of the rectal wall with or without protrusion through the anus.[27] Partial rectal prolapse, or prolapse of only the rectal mucosa, is most frequently encountered in children between the ages of 1 and 5, and in the elderly. Partial prolapse is believed to be caused by an abnormality in the attachment of the mucosa to the submucosal layer. Straining may produce both partial and complete prolapse. Partial prolapse creates a protruding mass with radiating furrows (like the spokes on a wheel) and associated hemorrhoids.[27] True procidentia (full-thickness rectal prolapse) creates circular furrows.[26]

The initial treatment of partial prolapse is removal of contributing factors such as colon polyps, diarrhea, constipation, or laxative use. In infants the prolapse should be manually reduced following each defecation, with gauze placed over the anus, and the buttocks then taped together.[27] As the child grows older, the partial prolapse often decreases in size and frequency until it subsides altogether. If additional intervention is necessary, injection sclerotherapy, rubber band ligation, or surgical hemorrhoidectomy may be beneficial.

In adults, complete rectal prolapse is more common in older women. Multiparity and obstetrical trauma to the anal sphincter may predispose to this increase in women. The majority of adults present with the protruding rectal tissue, although bleeding, mucous discharge, and pain may be reported. The treatment for procidentia (complete prolapse) is surgical. There are many operations used for this condition, and all can result in some degree of incontinence. About 40% of the elderly who undergo abdominal proctopexy do not regain continence.[27]

Pruritus Ani

Pruritus ani is the symptom complex consisting of intense itching and burning discomfort of the perianal skin.[28] The itching and subsequent scratching can lead to skin breakdown, maceration, weeping, and superinfection. Itching is most common after a bowel movement or just before falling asleep. Multiple causes exist for pruritus ani, and attempts should be made to identify the specific cause and institute specific treatment[16,28–30] (Table 11.3). Patients with pruritus ani are generally healthy, vigorous men (4:1 male/female ratio) aged 20 to 50 years.[16,28]

Table 11.3. **Conditions Associated with Pruritus Ani**

Systemic illness
Diabetes mellitus
Hyperbilirubinemia
Leukemia
Aplastic anemia
Thyroid disease
Mechanical factors
Chronic diarrhea
Chronic constipation
Anal incontinence
Soaps, deodorants, perfumes
Hemorrhoids producing leakage
Prolapsed hemorrhoids
Alcohol-based anal wipes
Rectal prolapse
Anal papilloma
Anal fissure
Anal fistula
Skin sensitivity from foods
Tomatoes
Caffeinated beverages
Beer
Citrus products
Milk products
Medications
Colchicine
Quinidine
Dermatologic conditions
Psoriasis
Seborrheic dermatitis
Intertrigo
Neurodermatitis
Bowen's disease
Atopic dermatitis
Lichen planus
Lichen sclerosis
Contact dermatitis
Infections
Erythrasma (*Corynebacterium*)
Intertrigo (*Candida*)
Herpes simplex virus
Human papillomavirus
Pinworms (*Enterobius*)
Scabies
Local bacterial abscess
Gonorrhea
Syphilis

A complete skin examination with focus on the mouth, scalp, and nails may provide evidence for a coexisting dermatologic condition (see Chapter 12). The perianal tissues should be closely inspected for primary perianal pathology. Pinworms and *Candida* infections are the most common infections associated with pruritus ani.[30] Unfortunately, in most patients there is no demonstrable cause.[16]

Patients should be educated about proper perineal hygiene. Soaps and talcum powders should be avoided, and patients should use white, undyed, unscented toilet tissue to limit allergic skin reactions. Excessive anal wiping is discouraged as it may produce skin lichenification.[30] Loosely fitting, dry cotton undergarments should be worn. Men who sweat excessively during the day can be encouraged to change their underwear at midday to limit moisture on the skin.

Pruritus ani can be difficult to treat. An empiric trial of a combination steroid and antifungal cream often is recommended but may not be successful.[29] Limited symptomatic relief may be gained from the use of antihistamines.[29] Additional treatment recommendations appear in Table 11.4. Dermatologic referral can be considered for refractory cases.

Infectious Proctitis

Proctitis describes an inflammation limited to the distal 10 cm of the rectum.[31–35] Infectious proctitis usually is caused by sexually transmitted diseases such as *Neisseria gonorrhoeae* and *Chlamydia trachomatis.*[23] Proctitis is considered when patients complain of rectal discomfort, tenesmus, rectal discharge, and constipation.[23] The anorectal mucosa may appear red and friable, and a mucopurulent discharge often is noted.

Table 11.4. **Treatment Guidelines for Patients with Pruritus Ani**

Cleanse perianal tissues following defecation with water
Avoid applying soaps or vigorous scrubbing to tissues
Dry tissues with patting of cotton towel or hair dryer
Apply a thin cotton pledget dusted with unscented cornstarch between bowel movements
Consume high-fiber diet to regulate bowel movements
Eliminate foods that promote itching such as tomatoes, chocolate, nuts, citrus fruits, colas, coffee, tea, beer
Avoid topical medications as they create irritation
Use 1% hydrocortisone cream sparingly for itching
Systemic antihistamines may relieve itching at bedtime

Gonorrheal proctitis is most common in homosexual men. Rectal gonorrhea in women usually results in spread from the genital tract, although 6% of women with rectal involvement are culture-negative from the cervix.[23] The majority of infected individuals are asymptomatic.[25,36,37] The ability to express pus from the anal crypts is highly suggestive of gonorrhea.[37] Nearly one half of rectal swabs may be falsely negative for gonorrhea, and empiric treatment is warranted when a high suspicion for the disease exists. Intramuscular ceftriaxone has replaced procaine penicillin G as the recommended treatment due to increasing penicillinase-producing *N. gonorrhoeae*.[23,31] Reculturing is recommended in 1 to 2 months, as treatment failure rates may be as high as 35%.[23]

Chlamydia trachomatis is recovered in 15% of asymptomatic homosexual men.[23] Because of the high rate of coexisting disease, all persons with gonorrhea should be treated for presumed *Chlamydia* infection (Table 11.5). Lympho-granuloma venereum (LGV), also caused by *C. trachomatis* serovars, can produce proctocolitis, inguinal adenopathy, and fistulas.[31] The sigmoidoscopic appearance with LGV is usually more severe, whereas *Chlamydia* proctitis usually produces a nonspecific erythema of the mucosa.

Viral infections can cause proctitis. Herpes simplex virus may produce vesicles, ulcers, itching, fever, sacral paresthesias, urinary re-

Table 11.5. **Commonly Recommended Treatments for Infectious Proctitis**

Causative organism	Treatment
Neisseria gonorrhoeae[a]	Ceftriaxone 250 mg IM (single dose)
Chlamydia trachomatis	Doxycycline 100 mg po two times daily for 7 days
Herpes simplex virus	Acyclovir 800–1600 mg/day po for 10 days
Syphilis (*Treponema pallidum*)	Benzathine penicillin G 2.4 million units IM
Entamoeba histolytica	Metronidazole 750 mg po three times daily for 10 days
Shigella species	Trimethoprim-sulfamethoxazole DS po two times daily for 7 days
Campylobacter jejuni	Erythromycin 500 mg po four times daily for 7 days

[a]Consider empiric treatment with doxycycline because of the high rate of concomitant infection with *Chlamydia trachomatis*.

tention, and impotence.[23] The anoscopic findings include erythema, diffuse ulcerations, and occasional pustules. Acyclovir can be used to shorten the clinical course or decrease shedding (400 mg five times daily for 10 days) or used daily (400 mg twice a day) to prevent recurrences.[32]

Syphilis proctitis generally produces multiple painless chancres in the perianal or anal area. Inguinal adenopathy may be present, and ulcers may be painful if secondarily infected.[23] Darkfield examination of scrapings or serologic testing can be used to document the infection. Follow-up serology is recommended 3 and 6 months following treatment.

Hidradenitis Suppurativa

Hidradenitis suppurativa is a chronic, inflammatory disease of the apocrine sweat glands of the skin.[17] Hidradenitis can develop in the perianal tissues, and often the skin changes are mistaken for perianal fistulas. Hidradenitis develops after puberty and is more common in individuals with oily skin. The patient may develop firm nodules that can coalesce into bands or plaques. Induration, drainage, and tenderness commonly are seen. Surgical treatment includes complete excision of the affected skin in single or multiple stages.[17]

Condyloma Acuminatum

Anal condyloma are caused by the human papillomavirus (HPV), usually types 6 and 11.[33] Anal warts appear to be most common in young men, especially those engaging in anal intercourse.[31] Women with anal warts often have coexisting warts on the cervix and labia. Smoking and alterations in immune system function [poor nutrition, human immunodeficiency virus (HIV) disease, severe allergies] may predispose to HPV infection.

Anal warts often are multiple and extend from the anal skin into the anal canal. Anoscopy is always indicated to evaluate the extent of disease.[34] Most patients exhibit only slight symptoms, such as irritation, moisture on the tissues, and occasional bleeding with defecation. Malignant degeneration of the underlying tissues can occur, especially in patients with HIV disease.[35] The goal of therapy is amelioration of signs and symptoms—not the eradication of HPV.[31]

The presence of anogenital warts in children incites high emotional response, and management is controversial.[34] While up to half of these children have been sexually abused, many acquire the infection by vertical transmission at birth. Assessment by a multidisciplinary team with set procedures for the consideration of abuse is appropriate.[34]

Multiple therapies exist for anogenital condylomas.[31,33] Podophyllin (25% concentration, applied for 5 to 10 minutes) and bichloracetic acid are topical agents applied weekly to destroy the warts.[32] Bichloracetic acid can be used in the anal canal,[32] an important consideration as up to 70% of homosexual men with external warts will have lesions up to the dentate line.[34] Both treatments can produce significant local skin irritation. Cryotherapy also is an effective destructive treatment but often is painful when applied to the perianal tissues.

Scissors excision following local anesthesia, and electrosurgical excision and destruction are effective techniques for removing condyloma.[32] The smoke plume generated at electrosurgery carries HPV particles, and an appropriate smoke evacuator should be used to protect both the patient and health care providers. Intralesional recombinant interferon-α is approved for treatment of condyloma (1 million units injected into each lesion three times a week on alternate days for 3 weeks).[32] Historically, application of topical 5-fluorouracil (5-FU) cream has been used to eliminate perianal warts. The potential for severe local skin effects has all but eliminated use of 5-FU cream.

Anal Carcinoma

Five types of malignant epithelial growths may develop in the anal region. Adenocarcinomas are the most common malignancies in the region, and most descend from the rectum above.[17] Between 2% and 6% of all anal cancers are squamous cell carcinomas.[17] Squamous cell carcinomas of the anal canal, historically aggressive tumors, are treated with irradiation, chemotherapy, and abdominopelvic resection.[17] Malignant melanomas, basal cell carcinomas, and primary adenocarcinomas of the anal canal are encountered much less commonly.

References

1. Pemberton JH. Anatomy and physiology of the anus and rectum. In: Zuidema GD, ed. Shackelford's surgery of the alimentary tract, 3rd ed. Philadelphia: WB Saunders, 1991;242–74.
2. Leibach JR, Cerda JJ. Hemorrhoids: modern treatment methods. Hosp Med 1991;27:53–68.
3. Dennison AR, Wherry DC, Morris DL. Hemorrhoids: nonoperative management. Surg Clin North Am 1988;68:1401–9.

4. Smith LE. Anal hemorrhoids. Neth J Med 1990;37:S22–32.
5. Schussman LC, Lutz LJ. Outpatient management of hemorrhoids. Prim Care 1986;13:527–41.
6. Medich DS, Fazio VW. Hemorrhoids, anal fissure, and carcinoma of the colon, rectum, and anus during pregnancy. Surg Clin North Am 1995;75:77–88.
7. Thomson WHF. The nature of haemorrhoids. Br J Surg 1975;62:542–52.
8. Stahl TJ. Office management of common anorectal problems. Postgrad Med 1992;92:141–51.
9. Zuber TJ. Anorectal disease and hemorrhoids. In: Taylor RB, ed. Manual of family practice. Boston: Little, Brown, 1997;381–4.
10. Ferguson EF. Alternatives in the treatment of hemorrhoidal disease. South Med J 1988;81:606–10.
11. Russel TR, Donohue JH. Hemorrhoidal banding: a warning. Dis Colon Rectum 1985;28:291–3.
12. Senagore A, Mazier WP, Luchtefeld MA, MacKeigan JM, Wengert T. Treatment of advanced hemorrhoidal disease: a prospective, randomized comparison of cold scalpel vs. contact Nd:YAG laser. Dis Colon Rectum 1993;36:1042–9.
13. Friend WG. External hemorrhoids. Med Times 1988;116:108–9.
14. Buls JG. Excision of thrombosed external hemorrhoids. Hosp Med 1994;30:39–42.
15. Grosz CR. A surgical treatment of thrombosed external hemorrhoids. Dis Colon Rectum 1990;33:249–50.
16. Mazier WP. Hemorrhoids, fissures, and pruritus ani. Surg Clin North Am 1994;74:1277–92.
17. Goligher J, Duthie H, Nixon H. Surgery of the anus rectum and colon, 5th ed. London: Baillière, 1984.
18. Gorfine SR. Treatment of benign anal disease with topical nitroglycerin. Dis Colon Rectum 1995;38:453–7.
19. Madoff RD. Pharmacologic therapy for anal fissure [editorial]. N Engl J Med 1998;338:257–9.
20. Carapeti EA, Kamm MA, McDonald PJ, Chadwick SJD, Melville D, Phillips RKS. Randomized controlled trial shows that glyceryl trinitrate heals anal fissures, higher doses are not more effective, and there is a high recurrence rate. Gut 1999;44:727–30.
21. Brisinda G, Maria G, Bentivoglio AR, Cassetta E, Gui D, Albanese A. A comparison of injections of botulinum toxin and topical nitroglycerin ointment for the treatment of chronic anal fissure. N Engl J Med 1999;341:65–9.
22. Minguez M, Melo F, Espi A, et al. Therapeutic effects of different doses of botulinum toxin in chronic anal fissure. Dis Colon Rectum 1999;42:1016–21.
23. Bassford T. Treatment of common anorectal disorders. Am Fam Physician 1992;45:1787–94.
24. Toglia MR. Anal incontinence: an underrecognized, undertreated problem. Female Patient 1996;21:17–30.
25. Whitehead WE, Wald A, Diamant NE, Enck P, Pemberton JH, Rao SS. Functional disorders of the anus and rectum. Gut 1999;45(suppl II):II55–9.

26. Knight AL. Fecal impaction. In: Rakel RE, ed. Saunders manual of medical practice. Philadelphia: WB Saunders, 1996;259–60.
27. Abcarian H. Prolapse and procidentia. In: Zuidema GD, ed. Shackelford's surgery of the alimentary tract, 3rd ed. Philadelphia: WB Saunders, 1991;331–48.
28. Dailey TH. Pruritus ani. In: Zuidema GD, ed. Shackelford's surgery of the alimentary tract, 3rd ed. Philadelphia: WB Saunders, 1991;281–5.
29. Zellis S, Pincus SH. Pruritus ani and vulvae. In: Rakel RE, ed. Conn's current therapy 1996. Philadelphia: WB Saunders, 1996;815–6.
30. Aucoin EJ. Pruritus ani: practical therapy for persistent itching. Postgrad Med 1987;82:76–80.
31. Centers for Disease Control and Prevention. 1993 Sexually transmitted diseases treatment guidelines. MMWR 1993;42(RR-14):1–102.
32. Modesto VL, Gottesman L. Sexually transmitted diseases and anal manifestations of AIDS. Surg Clin North Am 1994;74:1433–64.
33. Bonnez W, Reichman RC. Papillomaviruses. In: Mandell GL, Bennett JE, Dolin R, eds. Mandell, Douglas and Bennett's principles and practices of infectious diseases, 4th ed. New York: Churchill Livingstone, 1995;1387–400.
34. Von Krogh G, Gross G. Anogenital warts. Clin Dermatol 1997;15:355–68.
35. Palefsky JM. Anal cancer and its precursors: an HIV-related disease. Hosp Physician 1993;Jan:35–42.
36. Toglia MR. Pathophysiology of anorectal dysfunction. Obstet Gynecol Clin North Am 1998;25:771–81.
37. Janicke DM, Pundt MR. Anorectal disorders. Emerg Med Clin North Am 1996;14:757–88.

12
Common Dermatoses

Daniel J. Van Durme

Acne Vulgaris

Acne is the most common dermatologic condition presenting to the family physician's office. There are an estimated 40 to 50 million people in the United States affected with acne, including about 85% of all adolescents between the ages of 12 and 25.[1] It can present with a wide range of severity and may be the source of significant emotional and psychological, as well as physical, scarring. As adolescents pass through puberty, and develop their self-image, the physical appearance of the skin can be critically important. Despite many effective treatments for this disorder, patients (and their parents) often view acne as a normal part of development and do not seek treatment. The importance of early treatment to prevent the physical and emotional scars cannot be overemphasized.

The multifactorial pathogenesis of acne is important to understand, as most treatments are not curative but rather are directed at disrupting selected aspects of development. Acne begins with abnormalities in the pilosebaceous unit. There are four key elements involved in acne development: (1) keratinization abnormalities, (2) increased sebum production, (3) bacterial proliferation, and (4) inflammation. Each may play a greater or lesser role and manifests as a different type or presentation of acne. Initially, there is an abnormality of keratinization and increased sebum. Cohesive hyperkeratosis of the cells lining the pilosebaceous unit combines with increased sebum to block the follicular canal with "sticky" cells and thus a microcomedo develops. This blocked canal leads to further buildup of sebum behind the plug. This sebum production can be increased by androgens and other factors as well. The plugged pilose-baceous unit is seen as a closed comedone ("whitehead"), or as an open comedone ("blackhead") when the pore dilates and the fatty acids in the sebaceous plug become oxidized. The normal bacterial flora of the skin, especially *Proprionybacterium acnes*, proliferates in this plug and releases chemotactic factors drawing in leukocytes. The plug may also lead to rupture of the pilosebaceous unit under the skin, which in turn causes an influx of leukocytes. The resulting inflammation leads to the development of papular or pustular acne. This process can be marked and accompanied by hypertrophy of the entire pilosebaceous unit, leading to the formation of nodules and cysts. There are also factors that can aggravate or trigger acne, such as an increase in androgens during puberty, cosmetics, mechanical trauma, or medications.[2,3]

Diagnosis

Diagnosis is straightforward and is based on the finding of come-dones, papules, pustules, nodules, or cysts primarily on the face, back, shoulders, or chest, particularly in an adolescent patient. The pres-ence of comedones is considered a necessity for the proper diagno-sis of acne vulgaris. Without comedones, one must consider rosacea, steroid acne, or other acneiform dermatoses. It is important for choice of therapy and for long-term follow-up to describe and classify the patient's acne appropriately. Both the quantity and the type of lesions are noted. The number of lesions indicates whether the acne is mild, moderate, severe, or very severe (sometimes referred to as grades I–IV). The predominant type of lesion should also be noted (i.e., comedonal, papular, pustular, nodular, or cystic).[3] Thus a patient with hundreds of comedones on the face may have "very severe come-donal acne," whereas another patient may have only a few nodules and cysts and have "mild nodulocystic acne."

Management

Prior to pharmacologic management it is important to review and dis-pel some of the misperceptions that many patients (and parents) have about acne. This condition is not due to poor hygiene, nor are black-heads a result of "dirty pores." Aggressive and frequent scrubbing of the skin may actually aggravate the condition. Mild soaps should be used regularly, and the face should be washed gently and dried well prior to the application of topical medication. Several studies have failed to implicate diet as a significant contributor to acne,[4] and fatty foods and chocolate have not been found to be significant causative agents. Nevertheless, if patients are aware of something in their diet that triggers a flare-up, they should avoid it.

All patients should be taught that acne can be suppressed or controlled when medicines are used regularly, but that the initial therapy usually takes several weeks to show significant benefit. As the current lesions heal, the medications work to prevent the eruption of additional lesions. Typically, a noticeable response to medication is seen in about 6 weeks, and patients must be informed of this time lapse so they do not give up too soon. Some patients may have some initial worsening in the appearance of the skin when they first start treatment.

The treatment options for acne are based on several factors, including the predominant lesion and skin type, the distribution of lesions, individual patient preferences, and some trial and error. Benzoyl peroxide has both antibacterial and mild comedolytic activity and serves as the foundation of most acne therapy. This agent is available as cleansing liquids and bars and as gels or creams, with strengths ranging from 2.5% to 10%. The increase in strength increases the drying (and often the irritation) of the skin. It does not provide additional antibacterial activity. This agent can be used once or twice daily as basic therapy in most patients, although 1% to 2% of patients may have a contact allergy to it.[2]

Because all acne starts with some degree of keratinization abnormality and microcomedone formation, it is prudent to start with a comedolytic agent. Currently, the most effective agents are the topical retinoids—tretinoin (Retin-A, Avita), adapalene (Differin), and tazarotene (Tazorac). They are generally started at the lowest dose possible and thinly applied every night. Mild erythema and irritation are common at first. If they are severe, the frequency can be decreased to three times per week or less, and then slowly increased to every night. The strength of the preparation can also be gradually increased as needed and as tolerated over several weeks to months. Patients should be warned about some degree of photosensitivity with tretinoin and should use sun blocks as needed. Tazarotene is in pregnancy category X and must be avoided in pregnant women due to potential teratogenic effects. If benzoyl peroxide is also used, it is crucial to separate the application of these compounds by several hours. When applied close together, these preparations cause more irritation to the skin while inactivating each other, rendering treatment ineffective.

Antibiotics are recommended for papular or pustular (papulopustular) acne. They act by decreasing the proliferation of *P. acnes* and by inactivating the neutrophil chemotactic factors released during the inflammatory process. Topical agents include erythromycin (A/T/S 2%, Erycette solution), clindamycin (Cleocin T), tetracycline (Topicycline), and sodium sulfacetamide with sulfur (Novacet, Sulfacet-R). These agents are available in a variety of delivery vehicles and are applied once (sometimes twice) a day in conjunction with benzoyl peroxide. With both topical and oral antibiotics, some degree of trial and error is necessary. Some patients respond well to clindamycin, whereas another patient may respond only to erythromycin. Azelaic acid (Azelex) topical cream has been Food and Drug Administration (FDA) approved since 1996 for inflammatory acne and has some antibacterial and comedolytic activity. It should be used with caution in patients with a dark complexion, due to potential hypopigmentation. Additionally, benzoyl peroxide is available as a combination gel with erythromycin (Benzamycin) or with clindamycin (BenzaClin) and can be convenient and effective, but somewhat expensive.

Oral antibiotics are indicated for patients with severe or widespread papulopustular acne or patients with difficulty reaching the affected areas on their body (i.e., on the back). The most commonly used oral antibiotics are tetracycline and erythromycin, which are started at 1 g/day in divided doses. Tetracycline patients are warned of the photosensitivity side effect and advised to take the medicine on an empty stomach, without dairy products. Erythromycin patients should be warned of potential gastrointestinal (GI) upset. Other options for oral medications are doxycycline (50–100 mg twice a day), minocycline (50–100 mg twice a day), and occasionally trimethoprim-sulfamethoxazole (Bactrim DS or Septra DS 1 tablet once daily) for the refractory cases. As the acne improves, the dose of the oral medications can often be gradually decreased to about one-half the original dose for long-term maintenance therapy.[5,6]

Oral contraceptives have also been shown to have substantial benefits in many young women with acne. The non-androgenic progestins, norgestimate (Ortho-Cyclen, Ortho-TriCyclen) or desogestrel (Ortho-Cept, Desogen) should be used, and may take 2 to 4 months to show benefit.[6,7]

Nodulocystic acne requires initial therapy with benzoyl peroxide, tretinoin, and antibiotics. If these agents fail to control the acne adequately, oral isotretinoin (Accutane) may be used. This agent has been extremely effective in decreasing the production of sebum and shrinking the hypertrophied sebaceous glands of nodulocystic acne. In most patients it induces a remission for many months or cures the condition. If lesions remain, they are usually more susceptible to conventional therapy as described above. Accutane treatment consists of a 16- to 20-week course at 0.5 to 2.0 mg/kg/day. Although this medicine can be profoundly effective, it has "black box" warnings about its teratogenicity and its association with pseudotumor cerebri. There are also numerous less severe side effects, including xerosis, cheilitis, epistaxis, myalgias, arthralgias, elevated liver enzymes, and others. Liver function tests, triglyceride levels, and complete blood counts should be frequently monitored. The highly teratogenic potential must be made clear to all female patients, and this medication must be used with extreme caution in all women with childbearing potential. Patient selection guidelines for women include (negative) serum pregnancy tests before starting, maintenance of two highly effective methods of contraception throughout therapy and for 1 to 2 months after therapy, and signed informed consent by the patient.[7,8]

Atopic Dermatitis

Atopic dermatitis (AD) is a common, chronic, relapsing skin condition with an estimated incidence of 10% in the United States. It usually arises during childhood, with about 85% of patients developing it during the first 5 years of life.[9] The disease presents with severe pruritus, followed by various morphologic features. It has been described as "the itch that rashes." Although AD can be found as an isolated illness in some individuals, it is often a manifestation of the multisystemic process of atopy, which includes asthma, allergic rhinitis, and atopic dermatitis. A family or personal history of atopy can be a key element in making the diagnosis.

While there are questions as to the specifics of the role of the immune system and allergies in AD, there is some type of abnormality in the cell-mediated immune system (a T-cell defect) in these patients. They have an increased suscepti-bility to cutaneous viral (and fungal) infections, especially herpes simplex, molluscum contagiosum, and papillomavirus.[10,11] However, even though about 80% of patients with AD have an elevated immunoglobulin E (IgE) level, there is not enough evidence to conclude what specific role allergies play in the development of this disease.[12,13] Thus even though many people are under the misperception that their skin is allergic to just about everything, they should be taught that the process is not a true allergy but rather a reaction of genetically abnormal skin to environmental stressors.

The eruption is eczematous and usually symmetric. It is erythematous, may have papules and plaques, and often has secondary changes of excoriations and lichenification. The persistent excoria-

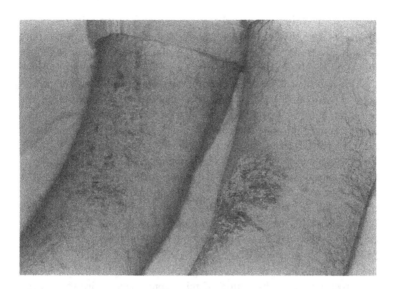

Fig. 12.1. Atopic dermatitis in the popliteal fossae.

tions can lead to secondary bacterial infection, which may be noted by more exudative and crusting lesions. In infants and children, AD is commonly seen on the face and the extensor areas, whereas in older children and adults it is more commonly seen in flexural areas of the popliteal and antecubital fossae and the neck and wrists (Fig. 12.1). Patients with AD may also have numerous other features including generalized xerosis, cheilitis, hand dermatitis, palmar hyperlinearity, and sensitivity to wool and lipid solvents (e.g., lanolin).[9,10]

Treatment of atopic dermatitis begins with attempts at moisturizing the skin. Bathing is done only when necessary and then with cool or tepid water and a mild soap (e.g., Dove or Purpose) or a soap substitute (e.g., Cetaphil). Immediately after bathing and gently patting the skin dry, an emollient is applied to the skin to help seal in the moisture. This emollient should have no fragrances, no alcohol, and no lanolin (e.g., Aquaphor, Keri lotion, Lubriderm) and should be used daily to maintain well-lubricated skin. If the affected areas are particularly severe in an acute outbreak, wet dressings with aluminum acetate solution (Burow's solution) can be applied two or three times daily. If the affected area has dry, noninflamed skin, a moisturizer with lactic acid (e.g., Lac-Hydrin) can be of such help that steroids can be avoided.

Controlling the intense pruritus is important. Keeping the nails trimmed short, and the use of mittens at night can decrease the excoriations in children. Topical steroids can control the inflammatory process. Generally the lowest possible potency should be used, but often high-potency creams may be needed on lichenified areas. In infants and children, one can often maintain good control with 0.25% to 2.5% hydrocortisone cream or ointment, applied two or three times a day. For more severe cases and in adults, 0.1% triamcinolone cream or ointment (or an equivalent-strength steroid) may be needed. Only rarely should fluorinated steroid preparations be used. While the underlying pathogenesis and the pruritus of AD are not primarily histamine mediated, many authors recommend the use of antihistamines that can be adjusted and titrated to balance the antipruritic effect with any potential sedating effects.[9–11] The more traditionally sedating antihistamines such as diphenhydramine (Benadryl) or hydroxyzine (Atarax, Vistaril) can be used at night and loratadine (Claritin) or cetirizine (Zyrtec) can be used during the day. Doxepin hydrochloride 5% cream (Zonalon) has both H_1 and H_2 blocking effects and may help to control pruritus without the problems of long-term topical steroid use; however, absorption of this agent leads to drowsiness in some patients, particularly if a large amount of the skin is treated. Tacrolimus ointment (Protopic) is an immunomodulating agent that was FDA approved for AD in 2001. It works similarly to cyclosporine and has been shown to be safe and effective for both long- and short-term use in AD.[14]

If the AD suddenly becomes much worse, development of a secondary infection or a possible contact dermatitis must be considered. If there is secondary infection, antibiotics directed at *Staphylococcus aureus* are used. Dicloxacillin, erythromycin, cephalexin, and topical mupirocin (Bactroban) are good choices. For patients prone to recurrent impetigo, it is reasonable to have a usual supply of mupirocin at home for any outbreaks. If these measures fail to provide adequate control, it is reasonable to pursue possible specific provocative factors such as foods, contact allergens or irritants, dust mites, molds, or possible psychological stressors.[9]

This condition can produce a great deal of anxiety and frustration in both patients and parents, and the stress can further aggravate the condition. Although psychological factors aggravate the condition, it is important to emphasize that the condition is not caused by "nerves." It is an inherited condition that can be aggravated by emotional stress. This supportive counseling for the patient and the family can be crucial. Furthermore, although affected children may appear "fragile," they are not, and they may desperately need some affectionate handling to help ease their own anxieties about their condition.[15]

Miliaria

Miliaria (heat rash) is a common condition resulting from the blockage of eccrine sweat glands. There is an inflammatory response to the sweat that leaks through the ruptured duct into the skin, and papular or vesicular lesions result. It usually occurs after repeated exposure to a hot and humid environment. Miliaria can occur at any age but is especially common in infants and children.[16]

One of the most common forms of miliaria is miliaria crystallina, in which the blockage occurs near the skin surface and the sweat collects below the stratum corneum. A thin-walled vesicle then develops, but there is little to no erythema. This situation is often seen in infants or bedridden patients and can be treated with cool compresses and good ventilation to control perspiration.

Miliaria rubra (prickly heat or heat rash) is more commonly seen in susceptible patients of any age group when exposed to sufficient heat. In this case the occlusion is at the intraepidermal section of the sweat duct. As a result there is more erythema, sometimes a red halo, or just diffuse erythema with papules and vesicles. Occasionally, the eruptions become pustular, resulting in miliaria pustulosa. There is usually more of a mild stinging or "prickly" sensation than real pruritus. The condition is self-limited but can be alleviated by cool wet to dry soaks. A low-strength steroid lotion (e.g., 0.025% or 0.1% triamcinolone lotion) is often helpful for alleviating the symptoms in these patients.[10]

Pityriasis Rosea

Pityriasis rosea (PR) is a benign, self-limited condition primarily found in patients between the ages of 10 and 35. The cause is unknown, but a viral etiology is suspected as some patients have a prodrome of a viral-like illness with malaise, low-grade fever, cough, and arthralgias; there is an increased incidence in the fall, winter, and spring.[17]

This disorder typically starts with a single, 2- to 10-cm, oval, papulosquamous, salmon-pink patch (or plaque) on the trunk or proximal upper extremity. This "herald patch" is followed by a generalized eruption of discrete, small, oval plaques on the trunk and proximal extremities, sparing the palms and soles and oral cavity. These plaques align their long axis with the skin lines, thus giving the rash a characteristic "Christmas tree" appearance (Fig. 12.2). The plaques often have a fine, tissue-like "collarette" scale at the edges.

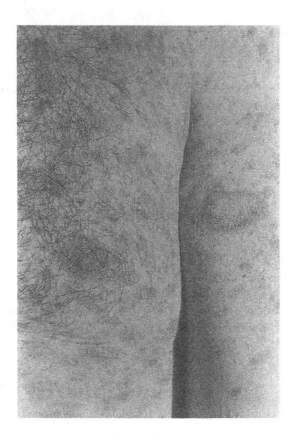

Fig. 12.2. Pityriasis rosea. (Note herald patch on arm.)

The differential diagnosis includes tinea corporis, as the initial herald patch can be confused with ringworm. The diffuse eruption of PR may resemble secondary syphilis but can often be distinguished by the sparing of the palms and soles in PR. It may also give the appearance of psoriasis (especially guttate psoriasis) but has much finer plaques that are not clustered on the extensor areas. Finally, the eruption may be confused with tinea versicolor. Skin scrapings for a potassium chloride (KOH) preparation should be strongly considered in any patient with apparent PR, as well as serologic testing for syphilis in any sexually active patient.

The management of PR is fairly easy. Pruritus is generally mild and can be controlled with oral antihistamines or topical low-potency steroid preparations. Patients can be reassured that the lesions will fade within about 6 weeks, but may last up to 10 weeks. They should be warned, however, that postinflammatory hypo- or hyperpigmentation (especially in those with more darkly pigmented skin) is possible.[17]

Psoriasis

Psoriasis is a chronic, recurrent disorder characterized by an inflammatory, scaling, hyperproliferative papulosquamous eruption. Lesions are well-defined plaques with a thick, adherent, silvery white scale. If the scale is removed, pinpoint bleeding can be seen (Auspitz's sign). Psoriasis occurs in about 1% to 3% of the worldwide population.[18] The etiology is unknown, although some genetic link is suspected, as one third of patients have a positive family history for the disease. It may start at any age, with the mean age of onset during the late twenties.[19]

Lesions most commonly occur on the extensor surfaces of the knees and elbows but are also typically seen on the scalp and the sacrum and can affect the palms and soles as well. The nails may show pitting, onycholysis, or brownish macules ("oil spots") under the nail plate. Finally, up to 20% of these patients may develop psoriatic arthritis, which can be severe, even crippling.[20]

Although psoriasis is usually not physically disabling and longevity is not affected, the patient's physical appearance can be profoundly affected and may cause significant psychological stress as the patient withdraws from social activities. Attention to the psychosocial implications of this chronic disease is crucial for every family physician.

The classic presentation, chronic plaque psoriasis or psoriasis vulgaris, demonstrates erythematous plaques and silvery adherent scales on elbows, knees (Fig. 12.3), scalp, or buttocks. It is usually easy to diagnose when in the classic form, but there are numerous morphologic variants. Discoid, guttate, erythrodermic, pustular, flexural (intertriginous), light-induced, and palmar-plantar psoriasis are among the many clinical presentations of this condition. The plaques may be confused with seborrheic or atopic dermatitis, and the guttate variant may resemble pityriasis rosea or secondary syphilis. If the diagnosis is unclear, referral to a dermatologist or a biopsy (read by a dermatopathologist, if possible) is in order.

The lesions often appear on areas subjected to trauma (Koebner phenomenon). Other precipitating factors include infections, particularly upper respiratory infections, and stress. Several drugs, partic-

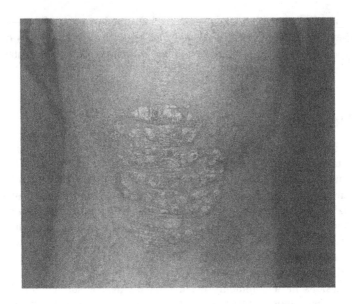

Fig. 12.3. Typical psoriatic plaque.

ularly lithium, beta-blockers, angiotensin-converting enzyme (ACE) inhibitors, and antimalarial agents are well known to trigger an outbreak or exacerbate existing psoriasis in some patients.[18,19] The nonsteroidal antiinflammatory drugs (NSAIDs) used for psoriatic arthritis may worsen the skin manifestations. Systemic corticosteroids can initially clear the psoriasis, but a "rebound phenomenon," or worsening of the lesions, even after slowly tapering the dose is common.

Management

Patients must understand that there is no cure for psoriasis. All treatments are suppressive (i.e., designed to control the manifestations, improve the cosmetic appearance for the patient, and, it is hoped, induce a remission). Therapy should start with liberal use of emollients and mild soaps. Moderate exposure to sunlight, while avoiding sunburn, can also improve the condition. After this start, treatment modalities are divided into topical agents and systemic therapies. The decision to use systemic agents is usually based on the percent of body surface area involved, with 20% often being used as the cutoff for changing to systemic treatment. In practice, however, the decision to use systemic therapy is based on the severity of the disease, the resistance to topical treatments, the availability of other agents, and a complex of social and psychological factors.[18–22] This decision is usually best made by an experienced dermatologist in consultation with the patient and the family physician.

Keratolytic preparations such as those with salicylic acid (Keralyt gel) or urea-based (Lac-Hydrin) can soften plaques and increase the efficacy of other topical agents. With the exception of emollients, the topical treatments for chronic plaque psoriasis should be applied to the lesions only and not the surrounding skin. It should be carefully explained to the patient that the medications that stop the overgrowth of the psoriatic skin have side effects on the normal surrounding skin and application should be done carefully.

Topical steroid preparations are a typical starting point for psoriasis, and while they can provide prompt relief, it is often temporary. Tolerance to these agents is common (tachyphylaxis), and one must remain vigilant for the long-term side effects of thinning of the skin, hypopigmentation, striae, and telangiectasia. The lowest effective strength is used, always using caution with higher strengths on the face, groin, and intertriginous areas. Increased efficacy is seen when ointments are used under occlusion, but this practice can also lead to enough systemic absorption to suppress the pituitary-adrenal system.[20]

The topical agent calcipotriene 0.005% (Dovonex) has shown good results with mild to moderate plaque psoriasis. It is a derivative of vitamin D and works by inhibiting keratinocyte and fibroblast proliferation. It is available as a cream, ointment, or scalp solution and is applied as a thin layer twice a day with most improvement noted within 1 month. Side effects include itching or burning in 10% to 20% of patients and rare cases of hypercalcemia (<1%), particularly when large amounts are used (>100 g/week).[21]

Tazarotene (Tazorac) is a topical retinoid gel that inhibits epidermal proliferation and inflammation in psoriasis (and is also FDA approved for acne vulgaris). Tazarotene alone has shown only modest benefit and can often cause irritation. Optimal benefit from this agent is obtained by combining it with a medium-potency steroid, such that tazarotene is applied each night and the steroid is applied each morning. This drug must be avoided in pregnant women due to potential teratogenic effects.[21]

Chronic plaques can often be managed by using the antimitotic agents of anthralin or coal tar. Anthralin preparations (e.g., Anthra-Derm, Drithocreme, Dritho-Scalp) can be applied to thick plaques in the lowest dose possible for about 15 minutes a day and then showered off. Care must be taken to avoid the face, genitalia, and flexural areas. The duration and strength of the preparation is gradually increased as tolerated until irritation occurs. This preparation is messy and can stain normal skin, clothing, and bathroom fixtures. Coal tar preparations can be used alone or, more successfully, in combination with ultraviolet B (UVB) light therapy (Goeckerman regimen).[19] Coal tar may be found in both crude and refined preparations, such as bath preparations, gels, ointments, lotions, creams, solutions, soaps, and shampoos. In general, the treatment is similar to that with anthralin; progressively higher concentrations are used as needed until irritation or improvement results. The preparations are left on overnight, and staining can be a problem.

When systemic therapy is needed, treatment with ultraviolet (UV) light can be extremely effective. There are two basic regimens: One uses UVB (alone or with coal tar or anthralins) and the other uses UVA light therapy with oral psoralens (PUVA) therapy. The psoralen acts as a photosensitizer, and the UVA is administered in carefully measured amounts via a specially designed unit. Phototherapy and photochemotherapy can be expensive and carcinogenic. Thus they are administered only by an experienced dermatologist. Other systemic agents include the retinoid acitretin (Soriatane), methotrexate, etretinate (Tegison), and cyclosporine.[18–21] Due to the numerous side effects of these medicines, their use is generally best left to an experienced dermatologist and is beyond the scope of this text.

The lesions of psoriasis may disappear with treatment, but residual erythema, hypopigmentation, or hyperpigmentation is common. Patients must be instructed to continue treatment until there is near or complete resolution of the induration and not to always expect complete disappearance of the lesions.

Family and Community Issues

Proper patient and family education is crucial for managing the physical and psychosocial manifestations of this disease. The patient should be allowed to participate in the decision of which treatment modalities will be used and must be carefully instructed on the proper use of the one(s) chosen. The ongoing emotional support the family physician provides can help prevent the emotional scars that psoriasis may leave behind. The National Psoriasis Foundation (6600 SW 92nd, Suite 300, Portland, OR 97223; phone 800-723-9166, *www.psoriasis.org*) is a nonprofit organization dedicated to supporting research and education in this field. It provides newsletters and other educational material for patients and their families. A written prescription with the address and Web site can be one of the most effective long-term "treatments" for these patients.

Poison Ivy, Poison Oak, and Sumac (Rhus Dermatitis)

Plant-related contact dermatitis can be triggered by numerous plant compounds, but the most common allergen is the urishiol resin found in the genus *Toxicodendron* (formerly *Rhus*) containing the plants poison ivy, poison oak, and poison sumac. These three plants cause more allergic contact dermatitis than all other contact materials combined.[10] The oleoresin urishiol, which serves as the allergen (and rarely as a primary irritant), is located within all parts of the plant.[23]

The clinical presentation varies with the amount of the allergen and the patient's own degree of sensitivity. About 70% to 80% of Americans are mildly to moderately sensitive to the allergen, with about 10% to 15% at each end of the spectrum—either very sensitive or completely tolerant.[24] The eruption is erythematous with papules, wheals, and often vesicles. In severe cases, large bullae or diffuse urticarial hives are seen. The distribution is often linear or streak-like on exposed skin from either direct contact with the plant or by inadvertent spreading of the resin by the patient.

A history of exposure to the plant or to any significant activities outdoors helps in the diagnosis. It must be remembered, however, that the resin adheres to animal hair, clothing, and other objects and can then cling to the patient's skin after this indirect contact. Thus the patient may not be aware of any direct exposure. The thick, calloused skin on the hands often prevents eruption on the palms while the resin is transferred to another part of the body, where an eruption does occur. Outbreaks typically occur within 8 to 48 hours of the exposure. Alternatively, the initial exposure may sensitize the patient so the rash occurs a couple of weeks after exposure in response to the resin remaining on or in the skin.[23] The ability of the resin to remain on the skin (even after washing) and cause a later eruption has led to the mistaken belief that the fluid of the vesicles can cause spreading of the lesions.

Treatment begins with removal of any remaining allergen by thorough skin cleansing with soap and water as soon after exposure as possible. Rubbing (isopropyl) alcohol can be even more effective in dispersing the oily resin. Any clothing that may have come in contact with the plant should also be washed. If the affected area is small, and there is no significant vesicular formation, topical steroids (medium to high potency, such as triamcinolone 0.1–0.5%) are sufficient. The blisters can be relieved by frequent use of cool compresses with water or with Burow's solution (one packet or tablet of Domeboro in 1 pint of water). Oral antihistamines (e.g., diphenhydramine 25–50 mg or hydroxyzine 10–25 mg, four times a day) can help relieve the pruritus. If the outbreak is severe or widespread, or it involves the face and eyes, oral steroids may be needed. A tapering dose of prednisone (starting at 0.5–1.0 mg/kg/day) can be used over 5 to 7 days if the outbreak started a week or more after exposure. A longer, tapering course should be used (10–14 days) if treating an outbreak that started within 1 to 2 days of exposure. This regimen treats the lesions that are present and should suppress further development of lesions as the skin is sensitized.[24]

Prevention is best done by avoidance of the plants altogether or using clothing (that is then carefully removed to avoid rubbing the resin on the skin) as a barrier. The FDA has approved the first medication proved to prevent outbreak, bentoquatam (IvyBlock). This nonprescription lotion is applied before potential exposure and dries on the skin to form a protective barrier. This lotion does not irritate or sensitize the skin and provides 4 to 8 hours of protection. Desensitization attempts have not been successful and are not recommended.

Seborrheic Dermatitis

Seborrheic dermatitis, a chronic, recurrent scaling eruption, is common (incidence 3–5%) and typically occurs on the face, scalp, and the areas of the trunk where sebaceous glands are more prominent. It is usually seen in two age groups: infants during the first few months of life (may present as "cradle cap") and adults ages 30 to 60 (dandruff). It causes mild pruritus, is generally gradual in onset, and is fairly mild in its presentation. An increased incidence (up to 80%) has been described in patients with acquired immunodeficiency syndrome (AIDS), and these patients often present with a severe, persistent eruption.[25] The etiology is unknown, but there appears to be some link to the proliferation of the yeast *Pityrosporum ovale*, in the *Malassezia* genus. While this organism is present as normal flora for all people, the response of seborrheic dermatitis to antifungals agents strongly suggests a role for *P. ovale*.[26]

The lesions are scaling macules, papules, and plaques. They may be yellowish, thick and greasy, or sometimes white, dry, and flaky. Thick, more chronic lesions occasionally crust and then fissure and weep. Secondary bacterial infection leading to impetigo is not uncommon. The differential diagnosis includes atopic dermatitis, candidiasis, or a dermatophytosis. When the scalp is involved, the plaques are often confused with psoriasis, and the two conditions may overlap, referred to as seboriasis or sebopsoriasis. When the trunk is involved, the lesions may appear similar to those of pityriasis rosea.

Periodic use of shampoos containing selenium sulfide (Selsun, Selsun Blue), pyrithione zinc (Sebulon, Head and Shoulders), salicylic acid and sulfur combinations (Sebulex), or coal tar (Denorex, Neutrogena T-Gel) can be effective, not just on the scalp, but also on the trunk. The antifungal agent ketoconazole (Nizoral) is also available as a shampoo and can be highly effective. These shampoos are used two or three times a week and must be left on the skin (scalp) for about 5 to 10 minutes prior to rinsing. They are used alternating with regular soaps/shampoos as needed. This regimen may prevent the tachyphylaxis that can occur with daily use. After about 1 month the frequency of use can be decreased as tolerated to maintain control. Low-potency topical steroid creams or lotions such as 2.5% hydrocortisone or 0.01% fluocinolone (also available as a shampoo) can be used once or twice a day in the scalp or in other areas such as the face, groin, and chest. Topical ketoconazole cream (Nizoral) or terbinafine cream or spray (Lamisil) twice daily can also be helpful. Thick scales, such as may be found on the scalps of infants, can be gently scrubbed off with a soft toothbrush after soaking the area for 5 minutes with warm mineral oil or a salicylic acid shampoo. In severe and unresponsive cases, isotretinoin (Accutane) has been shown to be very effective in seborrheic dermatitis by markedly shrinking the size of the sebaceous glands and demonstrating some antiinflammatory effect. As compared to treatment for acne vulgaris, these patients often respond to lower doses (0.1 to 0.3 mg/kg/day) and shorter courses (4 weeks).[26] The same precautions, especially regarding pregnancy, that are described above must be observed.

Rosacea (Acne Rosacea)

A chronic facial dermatosis, acne rosacea typically appears in patients between the ages of 30 and 60. It is characterized by acneiform lesions such as papules, pustules, and occasionally nodules (Fig. 12.4). It is more common in those of Celtic, Scandinavian, or Northern European descent—those with fair skin who tend to flush easily. In addition to the facial flushing, generalized erythema, and telangiectasias, they may have moderate to severe sebaceous gland hyperplasia. Ocular manifestations such as conjunctivitis, blepharitis, and episcleritis can be found in more than half of the patients. Severe involvement of the nose can lead to soft tissue hypertrophy and rhinophyma. Otherwise, most lesions are on the forehead, cheeks, and

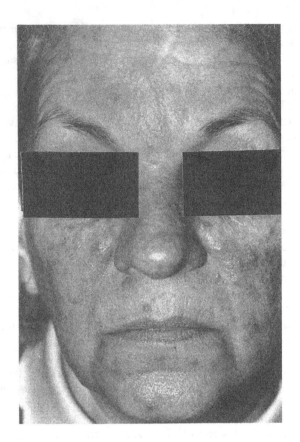

Fig. 12.4. Acne rosacea.

nose. The pathogenesis is unknown, but increasing evidence suggests that it is primarily a cutaneous vascular disorder that leads to lymphatic damage followed by edema, erythema, and finally papules and pustules.[27] Despite popular conception, alcohol is not known to play a causative role, but the vasodilatory effects of alcohol may make the condition appear worse. There is also some vasomotor instability in response to stress, sun exposure, hot liquids, and spicy foods, and these should be avoided.[28]

Treatment with oral erythromycin or tetracycline 1 g/day in divided doses or with minocycline or doxycycline at 50 to 100 mg twice a day can help alleviate both the facial and ocular manifestations of the disease. Response is variable, with some patients showing a prompt response followed by weeks or months of remission and others requiring long-term suppression with antibiotics. If long-term treatment is needed, the dose is titrated down to the minimal effective amount. Topical agents include clindamycin and erythromycin, but some of the better responses are seen with metronidazole 0.75% gel, lotion or cream (MetroGel, MetroLotion, Metrocream), or 1% cream (Noritate) in mild to moderate cases.[29] Topical sodium sulfacetamide and sulfur lotion is available in a unique preparation (Sulfacet-R) that includes a color blender for patients to add tint to the lotion to match their own skin coloration. This agent is popular with women in particular who may wish to hide the erythema and lesions. Oral metronidazole (Flagyl) may be used with caution in resistant cases. Topical tretinoin (Retin-A) and oral isotretinoin (Accutane) have shown promising results in patients with severe, refractory rosacea.[29–31]

Dyshidrotic Eczema (Pompholyx)

Dyshidrotic eczema, a recurrent eczematous dermatosis of the fingers, palms, and soles, is more common in the young population (under age 40) and typically presents with pruritic, often tiny, deep-seated vesicles. The etiology is unknown, but despite the name and the fact that many patients may have associated hyperhidrosis, it is not a disorder of sweat retention. Many of these patients have a history of atopic dermatitis, and it is considered a type of hand/foot eczema. Emotional stress plays a role in some cases, as does ingestion of certain allergens (e.g., nickel and chromate).[10]

The onset is typically abrupt and lasts a few weeks, but the disorder can become chronic and lead to fissuring and lichenification. Secondary bacterial infection can also occur. The vesicles are usually small but can be bullous and may give the appearance of tapioca. The most common site is the sides of the fingers in a cluster distribution (Fig. 12.5). The nails can also show involvement with dystrophic changes such as ridging, pitting, or thickening.

Controlling this disorder can be difficult and frustrating for the physician and patient alike. Attempts should be made to remove the inciting stressor whenever possible. Further treatment is similar to that for atopic dermatitis: Cool compresses may provide relief, and topical steroids can alleviate the inflammation and pruritus. It is one of the dermatoses in which high-potency fluorinated or halogenated steroids (in the ointment or gel formulation) are often needed to penetrate the thick stratum corneum of the hands. If secondary infection

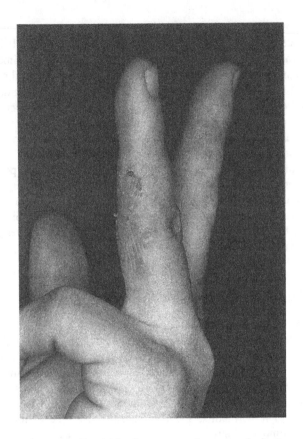

Fig. 12.5. Dyshidrotic eczema (or pompholyx).

is present, erythromycin or cephalexin can be helpful. Rarely, oral steroids may be needed, but these drugs are reserved for the more severe, recalcitrant cases.

Drug Eruptions

Rashes of various types are common reactions to medications. The dermatologic manifestations can be highly variable: maculopapular (or morbilliform) eruptions; urticaria; fixed, hyperpigmented lesions; photosensitivity reactions; vesicles and bullae; acneiform lesions; and generalized pruritus, among others. Serious and even life-threatening dermatologic reactions can occur as well, such as Stevens-Johnson syndrome, toxic epidermal necrolysis, hypersensitivity syndrome, and serum sickness.[31,32]

Definitively assigning a diagnosis of a particular eruption to a single agent can be difficult, as patients may take multiple medications, they may have coexistent illnesses, and the drug eruption may not manifest until the patient has been taking it for several days (sometimes weeks). Only when the eruption follows the administration a particular agent, resolves with removal of the agent, recurs with readministration, and other causes have been excluded can one say that the eruption is definitely due to a specific drug. Caution must be used prior to any rechallenge with an agent, and so readministration is often not recommended. Subsequently, many patients mistakenly believe they have dermatologic reactions or allergies to certain medications when their rash may have had nothing to do with their medication.

Table 12.1 lists several of the typical drug reactions to some of the more common drugs in clinical practice.[10,15,24,32–34] Treatment consists of stopping the offending (or suspected) medication. Topical low- to mid-potency steroids and oral antihistamines can relieve the pruritus that accompanies many eruptions.

Contact Dermatitis

Contact dermatitis is the clinical response of the skin to an external stimulant. It is an extremely common condition. Chemically caused dermatitis is responsible for an estimated 30% of all occupational illness.[35] The condition is such a problem with a wide variety of mechanisms of pathogenesis and potential products involved that an international journal, *Contact Dermatitis*, is devoted specifically to this topic. By suspecting virtually everything and anything and taking a thorough history, the family physician nevertheless should be able to diagnose and manage most of these patients.

While some authors describe several different subtypes of contact dermatitis, the two most common types are irritant contact dermatitis and allergic contact dermatitis. Morphologically and histologically, they can appear identical, and the difference to the clinician is more conceptual.[36] Irritant contact dermatitis accounts for the majority of cases of contact dermatitis, and results from a break in the skin's integrity and subsequent local absorption of an irritant. There is no true demonstrable allergen present. A single exposure can induce an inflammatory response if the agent is caustic enough or if there is a marked degree of exposure. Often the response is the re-

Table 12.1. **Common Reactions to Common Drugs**

Anaphylaxis	Maculopapular (morbilliform)	Serum sickness
Aspirin	Barbiturates	Aspirin
Sulfonamides	Isoniazid	Penicillin
NSAIDs	Phenothiazine	Sulfonamide
Serum (animal derived)	Sulfonamides and sulfonylureas	Urticaria
Penicillins	Lithium	Antibiotics
Fixed drug eruptions	NSAIDs	Opiates
Antibiotics— penicillins, sulfonamides,	Phenytoin	Blood products
tetracyclines	Thiazides	Radiocontrast agents
Phenolphthalein	Gentamicin	NSAIDs
Barbiturates	Penicillin compounds	Vesicular eruption
Dextromethorphan	Quinidine	Barbiturates
NSAIDs	Photosensitivity	Clonidine
Allopurinol	Carbamazepine	Naproxen
Lupus-like eruptions	Methotrexate	Sulfonamides
Hydralazine	Coal tar compounds	Captopril
Methyldopa	Oral contraceptives	Furosemide
Hydrochlorothiazide	Furosemide	Penicillin
Procainamide	NSAIDs	Cephalosporins
Isoniazid	Quinidine	Nalidixic acid
Quinidine	Tetracyclines	Piroxicam
	Griseofulvin	
	Phenothiazines	
	Sulfonamides and sulfonylureas	
	Thiazides	

NSAID = nonsteroidal antiinflammatory drug.

sult of prolonged exposure with repeated minor damage to the skin, such as in those who must wash their hands frequently. Common offending agents include soaps, industrial solvents, and topical medications (e.g., benzoyl peroxide, tretinoin, lindane, benzyl benzoate, anthralin).[37,38]

The second most common type is allergic contact dermatitis. It is a delayed hypersensitivity reaction that occurs after the body is sensitized to the offending agent. The reaction is thus often delayed somewhat from the time of exposure. The response varies depending on the individual's sensitivity, the amount and concentration of the allergen, and the degree of penetration. Poison ivy dermatitis is perhaps the most common form of allergic contact dermatitis (discussed earlier in the chapter). Other common offenders are nickel, fragrances, rubber chemicals, neomycin, thimerosal, parabens (found in sunscreens and lotions), and benzocaine (topical anesthetic).[36–38] Even topical steroid preparations have been reported to cause allergic contact dermatitis in some patients.[39]

Physical findings may be identical or may vary somewhat with different forms of contact dermatitis. The irritant type often causes an erythematous scaling eruption with a typically indistinct margin (Fig. 12.6), whereas the allergic type may cause more erythema, edema, vesicular formation, and weeping. The offending agent is often identified more by the shape of the eruption than the appearance of the skin (e.g., a watchband or the elastic band of some article of clothing).

Treatment is symptomatic after removal of the irritant or allergen. Cool compresses can provide relief from the pruritus, particularly if there is any weeping. Oral antihistamines may be needed along with topical steroids. Ointment compounds are recommended, as they are less irritating and sensitizing than most creams or lotions. The patient should avoid any topical preparations with benzocaine or other -caines, as they may aggravate the condition. In severe cases a tapering course of oral steroids over 1 to 2 weeks is necessary. Subacute and chronic cases may also be colonized with *Staphylococcus aureus*, and an oral antibiotic (e.g., dicloxacillin, erythromycin, or cephalexin) may speed resolution.

Avoidance of the irritant or allergen is sometimes difficult for patients. Their job may require some exposure, or it may be difficult to verify the specific agent. Testing with a commercially available patch test kit (T.R.U.E. Test Allergen Patch Test Panel) is the most reliable method of identifying a true allergic contact dermatitis and its causative agent.[39] This is particularly useful in developing a long-term plan of avoidance.

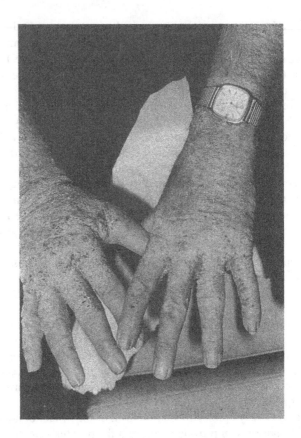

Fig. 12.6. Contact dermatitis, irritant type.

Urticaria

Urticaria, a common skin condition affecting about 20% of the population, is characterized by transient wheals or hives.[40] It is typically a type I immunologic reaction (mediated by IgE) but may be from physical or environmental exposure (pressure- or cold-induced). Urticaria can be acute (lasting less than 6 weeks) or chronic. Perhaps the most frustrating issue for the patient and physician faced with urticaria is that the underlying cause is often difficult to ascertain. In only about 20% of cases of chronic urticaria can the specific etiology be determined.[41,42]

A generalized eruption of pruritic wheals with erythema and localized edema and lesions lasting less than 24 hours establishes the diagnosis. Angioedema is a closely related process in which deeper tissues may be involved, particularly mucous membranes. Severe generalized urticaria can be a systemic illness leading to cardiac problems and even death.

One should search carefully to find the underlying etiology by doing a thorough comprehensive history and physical examination. Common causes include medications (antibiotics, NSAIDs, narcotics, radiocontrast dyes), illnesses (viral hepatitis, streptococcal, parasitic), connective tissue disorders (lupus, juvenile rheumatoid arthritis), endocrine disorders (hyper- or hypothyroidism), neoplastic disorders (lymphoma, leukemia, carcinoma), physical agents (pressure, cold, heat, exercise, menstruation), skin contacts (chemicals, fragrances, dyes, soaps, lotions, feathers, animal dander), insect bites and bee stings, foods (chocolate, shellfish, strawberries, nuts), and psychological stress.[10,15,40,41,43] The amount of laboratory work and other testing recommended can be highly variable and depends in part on the clinical utility of finding the underlying trigger(s). In general, an extensive workup is not advised during the first 6 weeks. Once the condition has persisted into chronic urticaria, a thorough history is as effective as an extensive and costly laboratory workup in finding the underlying cause.[40,44]

Treatment consists of avoidance of any known or suspected precipitant and the use of medications as needed for comfort. The H_1-blockers such as cetirizine (Zyrtec), loratadine (Claritin), diphenhydramine, or hydroxyzine can be used alone or in combination with an H_2-blocker such as cimetidine (Tagamet). Doxepin, a tricyclic antidepressant, can also be helpful at 25 mg once or twice a day. For severe, acute urticaria, a tapering dose of prednisone over 2 weeks can be helpful. Chronic urticaria may require a great deal of maintenance emotional support, as the condition can make normal activities difficult. Patients must be reassured, and medications may be needed on a long-term daily basis.

References

1. White GM Recent findings in the epidemiologic evidence, classification, and subtypes of acne vulgaris. J Am Acad Dermatol 1998;39:S34–7.
2. Russell JJ. Topical therapy for acne. Am Fam Physician 2000;61: 357–66.
3. Leyden JJ. New understandings of the pathogenesis of acne. J Am Acad Dermatol 1995;32:S15–25.
4. Rosenberg EW. Acne diet reconsidered. Arch Dermatol 1981;117: 193–5.

5. Johnson BA, Nunley JR. Use of systemic agents in the treatment of acne vulgaris. Am Fam Physician 2000;62:1823–30,1835–6.
6. Leyden JJ. Therapy for acne vulgaris. N Engl J Med 1997;336(16): 1156–62.
7. Thiboutot D. New treatments and therapeutic strategies for acne. Arch Fam Med 2000;9:179–83.
8. Van Durme DJ. Family physicians and Accutane. Am Fam Physician 2000;62:1772–7.
9. Kristal L, Klein PA. Atopic dermatitis in infants and children. An update. Pediatr Clin North Am 2000;47:877–95.
10. Habif TP. Clinical dermatology: a color guide to diagnosis and therapy, 3rd ed. St. Louis: Mosby-Year Book, 1996.
11. Fleischer AB. Atopic dermatitis. Perspectives on a manageable disease. Postgrad Med 1999;106:49–55.
12. Borirchanyavat K, Kurban AK. Atopic dermatitis. Clin Dermatol 2000; 18:649–55.
13. Halbert AR, Weston WL, Morelli JG. Atopic dermatitis: is it an allergic disease? J Am Acad Dermatol 1995;33:1008–18.
14. Leicht S, Hanggi M. Atopic dermatitis. Postgrad Med 2001;109(6): 119–27.
15. Goldstein BG, Goldstein AO. Practical dermatology, 2nd ed. St. Louis: Mosby-Year Book, 1997.
16. Feng E, Janniger CK. Miliaria. Cutis 1995;55:213–6.
17. Bjornberg A, Tenger E. Pityriasis rosea. In: Freedberg IM, Eisen AZ, Wolff K, et al, eds. Dermatology in general medicine, 5th ed. New York: McGraw-Hill, 1999;541–6.
18. Greaves MW, Weinstein GD. Treatment of psoriasis. N Engl J Med 1995;332:581–8.
19. Christophers E, Moreweitz U. Psoriasis. In: Freedberg IM, Eisen AZ, Wolff K, et al, eds. Dermatology in general medicine. 5th ed. New York: McGraw-Hill, 1999;495–522.
20. Linden KG. Weinstein GD. Psoriasis: current perspectives with an emphasis on treatment. Am J Med 1999;107:595–605.
21. Pardasani AG, Feldman SR, Clark AR. Treatment of psoriasis: an algorithm-based approach for primary care physicians. Am Fam Physician 2000;61:725–33,736.
22. American Academy of Dermatology. Committee on Guidelines of Care, Task Force on Psoriasis. Guidelines of care for psoriasis. J Am Acad Dermatol 1993;28:632–7.
23. Tanner TL. Rhus (Toxicodendron) dermatitis. Prim Care 2000;27:493–502.
24. Pariser RJ. Allergic and reactive dermatoses. Postgrad Med 1991;89:75–85.
25. Janniger CK, Schwartz RA. Seborrheic dermatitis. Am Fam Physician 1995;52:149–59.
26. Johnson BA, Nunley JR. Treatment of seborrheic dermatitis. Am Fam Physician 2000;61:2703–10, 2713–14.
27. Wilkin JK. Rosacea: pathophysiology and treatment. Arch Dermatol 1994;130:359–62.

28. Zuber TJ. Rosacea. Prim Care 2000;27:309–18.
29. Thiboutot DM. Acne and rosacea. New and emerging therapies. Dermatol Clin 2000;18:63–71.
30. Ertl GA, Levine N, Kligman AM. A comparison of the efficacy of topical tretinoin and low dose oral isotretinoin in rosacea. Arch Dermatol 1994;130:319–24.
31. Hirsch RJ, Weinberg JM. Rosacea 2000. Cutis 2000;66:125–8.
32. Roujeau JC, Stern RS. Severe adverse cutaneous reactions to drugs. N Engl J Med 1994;33:1272–85.
33. Manders SM. Serious and life-threatening drug eruptions. Am Fam Physician 1995;51:1865–72.
34. Crowson AN. Recent advances in the pathology of cutaneous drug eruptions. Dermatol Clin 1999;17:537–60.
35. Anonymous. Contact dermatitis and urticaria from environmental exposures: Agency for Toxic Substances and Diseases Registry. Am Fam Physician 1993;48:773–80.
36. Rietschel RL Comparison of allergic and irritant contact dermatitis. Immunol Allergy Clin North Am 1997;17:359–64.
37. Oxholm A, Maibach MI. Causes, diagnosis, and management of contact dermatitis. Compr Ther 1990;16:18–24.
38. Adams RM. Recent advances in contact dermatitis. Ann Allergy 1991; 67:552–66.
39. Belsito DV. The diagnostic evaluation, treatment, and prevention of allergic contact dermatitis in the new millennium. J Allergy Clin Immunol 2000;105:409–20.
40. Greaves MW. Chronic urticaria. N Engl J Med 1995;332:1767–72.
41. Beltrani VS. Allergic dermatoses. Med Clin North Am 1998;82:1105–33.
42. Huston DP, Bressler RB. Urticaria and angioedema. Med Clin North Am 1992;76:805–40.
43. Mahmood T. Urticaria. Am Fam Physician 1995;51:811–6.
44. Kozel MM, Mekkes JR, Bossuyt PM, Bos JD. The effectiveness of a history-based diagnostic approach in chronic urticaria and angioedema. Arch Dermatol 1998;134:1575–80.

13
Diabetes Mellitus

*Charles Kent Smith, John P. Sheehan,
and Margaret M. Ulchaker*

Diabetes mellitus (DM) affects 12 million to 15 million individuals
in the United States, incurring an immense cost in terms of morbidity and premature death. The most prevalent form, type 2 DM, previously called adult-onset DM, has racial preponderances, female
predilection, and strong associations with obesity. During the 1980s
there was a revolution in DM management with the advent of home
blood glucose monitoring devices, human insulin, and reliable laboratory markers of long-term glycemic control. Additionally, published national and international standards of care have been disseminated directly to patients and physicians, heightening the
importance of adequate care and glycemic control to minimize devastating long-term complications.[1,2] Table 13.1 describes diagnostic
criteria for diabetes mellitus, impaired glucose tolerance, and gestational diabetes.

Heightened clinical awareness of the genetics and predisposing
factors should foster early diagnosis and adequate metabolic control
of the type 2 patient. In contrast, the type 1 DM patient generally
presents with a more precipitous clinical picture of ketoacidosis. Declining islet cell secretory function is more gradual, however, and
can evolve over a 10-year period. Understanding the autoimmune nature of islet destruction has led to experimental protocols attempting
to interrupt this process. Occasionally, there is diagnostic confusion
owing to a lack of a family history, the absence of significant keto-
sis, and the absence of significant obesity and other diagnostic hall-

Table 13.1. **Diagnostic Criteria for Diabetes Mellitus, Impaired Glucose Tolerance, and Gestational Diabetes**

Nonpregnant adults

Criteria for diabetes mellitus: Diagnosis of diabetes mellitus in nonpregnant adults should be restricted to those who have one of the following:

Fasting plasma glucose ≥126 mg/dL. Fasting is defined as no caloric intake for at least 8 hours.

Symptoms of diabetes mellitus (such as polyuria, polydipsia, unexplained weight loss) coupled with a casual plasma glucose level of ≥200 mg/dL. Casual is defined as any time of day without regard to time interval since the last meal.

2-hour postprandial plasma glucose ≥200 mg/dL during an oral glucose tolerance test. The test should be performed by World Health Organization criteria using a glucose load containing the equivalent of 75 g anhydrous glucose dissolved in water.

Note: In the absence of unequivocal hyperglycemia with acute metabolic decompensation, these criteria should be confirmed by repeat testing on a second occasion. The oral glucose tolerance test is not recommended for routine clinical use.

Criterion for impaired glucose tolerance: 2-hour postprandial plasma glucose ≥140 mg/dL and ≤199 mg/dL during an oral glucose tolerance test. The test should be performed by World Health Organization criteria using a glucose load containing the equivalent of 75 g anhydrous glucose dissolved in water.

Pregnant women

Criteria for gestational diabetes: After an oral glucose load of 100 g, gestational diabetes is diagnosed if two plasma glucose values equal or exceed:

Fasting: 105 mg/dL
1 Hour: 190 mg/dL
2 Hour: 165 mg/dL
3 Hour: 145 mg/dL

Source: Clinical practice recommendations: 2001.[1]

marks. The measurement of C-peptide levels, islet cell antibodies, and glutamic acid decarboxylase (GAD) antibodies provides useful diagnostic clarification.[3] C-peptide is the fragment produced when proinsulin, produced by the islets of Langerhans, is cleaved to produce insulin. For every molecule of insulin produced, a molecule of C-peptide has to exist; therefore, C-peptide is a marker of endogenous insulin production. Measurement of a C-peptide level is very useful in documenting insulin secretory capacity in the insulin-treated individual, in whom an insulin level would measure both endogenous and exogenous insulin. Careful clinical follow-up can clarify evolving absolute insulin deficiency even in the absence of these laboratory markers.

Pathophysiology

Previously, type 1 DM was considered to be an acute event. Viral associations were invoked with regard to the seasonal trends in its incidence. However, patients can have markers of islet destruction in the form of islet cell antibodies for up to 10 years prior to the development of overt DM. Islet cell, insulin, and GAD autoantibodies, along with the loss of first-phase insulin secretion in response to an intravenous glucose tolerance test, are highly predictive of evolving type 1 DM.[4] Attempts to interrupt this autoimmune process with immunosuppressive agents have been tried with some encouraging results, but toxicity remains a concern. Insulin has been given to experimental animals that have autoimmune islet destruction without overt DM in an attempt to suppress the autoimmune process. A pilot study of 12 patients demonstrated exciting promise for clinical applicability of this approach in humans.[5] However a nationwide clinical trial of prophylactic insulin in individuals at high risk to develop type 1 DM disappointingly showed no effect on the rate of progression to type 1 DM. A group of investigators in Edmonton, Alberta, Canada have treated seven patients with type 1 DM with islet cell transplantation. These patients who are initially on triple immunosuppression therapy have normal ambient glucose levels. However, on intravenous glucose tolerance testing, they have impaired glucose tolerance. The key to islet cell transplantation is developing safe immunosuppressives or modifying the process to eliminate the need for immunosuppressives.[6]

In contrast, type 2 DM is associated with genetic predispositions, advancing age, obesity, and lack of physical exercise. The importance of caloric intake and energy expenditure has been clearly established.[7] Although type 2 DM is a syndrome of insulin resistance and islet secretory defects, in any given individual it is not possible to define the degree of insulin resistance versus secretory defects with any precision. The earliest metabolic defect found in first-degree relatives of individuals with type 2 DM is defective skeletal muscle glucose uptake with later increased insulin resistance at the level of the liver and resultant uncontrolled hepatic glucose output. The ensuing hyperglycemia can have a toxic effect called glucotoxicity on the islets, resulting in secondary secretory defects with declining insulin secretion and self-perpetuating hyperglycemia. Hyperglycemia may also downregulate glucose transporters. To become hyperglycemic, insulin secretion must be insufficient to overcome the insulin resistance; it has been estimated that insulin secretory capacity is reduced by 50% at the time of diagnosis with type 2 DM.[8] It is unclear whether secretory defects or insulin resistance is the primary defect even for type 2 DM. Patients may exhibit many abnormalities, including loss of first-phase insulin secretion and loss of the pulsatility of insulin secretion.[9–12] Additionally, both men and women tend to have abdominal obesity, which is associated with hyperinsulinemia and insulin resistance.[13] Type 2 DM is a syndrome not only of disordered glucose metabolism but also of lipid metabolism; many patients have a concurrent dyslipidemia manifesting elevations in serum triglycerides, depressions in high-density lipoprotein (HDL) cholesterol, and marginal increases in total cholesterol. This dyslipidemia results from uncontrolled hepatic very low density lipoprotein (VLDL) secretion and defective clearance of lipoprotein molecules. The associations of hyperinsulinemia and insulin resistance with essential hypertension have been documented[14] along with the marked tendency for patients with essential hypertension to develop DM and the converse—patients with type 2 DM developing essential hypertension. A central unifying hypothesis focuses on hyperinsulinemia and insulin resistance being primary metabolic aberrations that result not only in hyperglycemia but also hypertension and dyslipidemia. Thus our current understanding of type 2 DM and the cardiodysmetabolic syndrome, formerly known as syndrome X[15] (hyperinsulinemia, dyslipidemia, hypertension, and hyperglycemia) highlights the important issue not only of primary prevention of type 2 DM but also secondary prevention.

Importance of Glycemic Control

The relation between microvascular complications of DM and glycemic control has been debated for decades. Many studies suggested an association between poor long-term glycemic control and retinopathy, neuropathy, and nephropathy. Unfortunately, many of these studies were not randomized, and the role of genetic factors was unclear. However, positive trends with glycemic control had been described. Small human studies and several animal studies link sustained metabolic control to the prevention of complications. One study showed, however, that early poor control despite later good control results in diabetic complications.[16] The Diabetes Control and

Complications Trial (DCCT) in individuals with type 1 DM proved the profound impact of intensive therapy on reducing the risk of microvascular complications.[17] Decades of questions about the glucose hypothesis are therefore finally answered, with the obvious recommendation that most individuals with type 1 DM be treated with intensive therapy. A potential negative aspect of attempts to achieve optimum glycemic control by intensive insulin therapy is the potential for severe hypoglycemia. An educated and motivated patient working with a multidisciplinary health care team can significantly reduce the risk of this. Glycemic goals may need to be modified in the individual with poor hypoglycemia awareness. The United Kingdom Prospective Diabetes Study (UKPDS), a 20-year prospective study in type 2 DM, demonstrated that both intensive glycemic control and intensive blood pressure control reduced the risk of microvascular and macrovascular complications of DM.[18–20] Excellent metabolic control as defined by normal hemoglobin A_{1c} (HbA_{1c}) levels without significant hypoglycemia is an achievable goal.

Defining Control

The definition of DM control has varied. During the bygone era of urine testing, predominantly negative urine tests were indicative of good glycemic control. However, because blood glucose can be twice normal in the absence of glycosuria, urine glucose monitoring is now outmoded. Home blood glucose monitoring (HBGM) provides positive feedback of daily glycemic control to patients and physicians. Patients engaged in intensive insulin therapy can monitor themselves four to ten times per day and make adjustments in their regimen to optimize blood glucose control. The precision and accuracy of the home units has improved considerably, as has the simplicity and duration of the test. Some systems enable users to obtain the blood sample from the forearm. Each system has its inherent weaknesses and limitations in such areas as blood volume, timing, hematocrit, temperature, and humidity. It is important that patients adhere strictly to the manufacturers' guidelines because attention to proper calibrations, strip handling, and ongoing maintenance are critical. Minimally invasive HBGM is the wave of the future, with the Glucowatch Biographer being the first to reach market. The HbA_{1c}, the marker of long-term glycemic control, measures the degree of glycosylation of the A_{1c} subfraction of hemoglobin and reflects the average blood glucose over the preceding 60 to 90 days. It also allows for identification of possible falsification of or errors in HBGM results. It is a useful motivating tool for patients; it often becomes a perceived challenge to reduce the result within the constraints of hypoglycemia. The National Glycosylated Hemoglobin Standardization Program is responsible for standardizing and correlating various assays to the DCCT methodology.[21]

Hemoglobinopathies can skew HbA_{1c} results, and can be detected via inspection of the chromatograms in the laboratory. The American Diabetes Association recommends that the HbA_{1c} be performed at least two to four times per year in all patients. Given that the DCCT demonstrated a linear relation between the HbA_{1c} (all the way into the normal, non-diabetic range) and microvascular complication risk, the ideal is therefore normalization of the HbA_{a1c} within the constraints of hypoglycemia. In addition to markers of glycemic control, it is critical to monitor other clinical parameters. Annual lipid profiles are an integral part of overall DM care in view of the high prevalence of dyslipidemia especially in the patient with type 2 DM. In type 1 DM patients, lipid disturbances are uncommon unless patients are in poor glycemic control, have a familial dyslipidemia, or have renal insufficiency. Markers of nephropathy are also important to measure. The earliest marker, microalbuminuria, is not only a forerunner of overt clinical nephropathy but also a marker for greatly increased cardiovascular risk in both type 1 and type 2 patients.[22,23] Microalbuminuria can be conveniently measured in spot urine specimens or by overnight albumin excretion rates,[24] rather than the more cumbersome 24-hour urine collection.

Patient Education

Patient attention to management principles decidedly affects short-term metabolic control and ultimately has an impact on long-term complications. The interactions of patients with registered nurses and dietitians (preferably certified diabetes educators) are critical. The presence of family members and significant others during the educational sessions is vital to a successful outcome. Education must encompass a comprehensive understanding of the pathophysiology of DM and its complications and the importance of attaining and sustaining metabolic control. Accurate HBGM is critical; after initial instruction, periodic reassessment of performance technique helps to ensure continued accuracy. The results stored in the memory of most meters can be downloaded to a computer, via a meter-specific computer program. However, the traditional written glucose log actually provides more information when an educated, motivated patient records glucose results, times of day, medication administered, and notes regarding activity and other variables. Education must also focus on dietary principles. For individuals with diabetes, the current dietary recommendations are a diet containing at least 50% of the calories from carbohydrate, less than 30% fat, and 20% or less protein. Caloric requirements are based on ideal body weight (IBW)—not actual body weight. We calculate IBW by the Hamwi formula.[25]

Women
   100 pounds for 5 feet
   5 pounds for every additional inch
   Example: Woman 5'3" = 115 pounds IBW

Men
   106 pounds for 5 feet
   6 pounds for every additional inch
   Example: Man 5'8" = 154 pounds IBW

Based on anthropometric measures, 10% may be subtracted or added based on small body frame or large body frame, respectively.

   Basal caloric requirements then are as follows.

Woman 5'3": IBW = 115 pounds
115 × 10 kcal = 1150 kcal/day

Add 300 to 400 kcal/day for moderate to strenuous activity. Subtract 500 kcal/day for 1 pound per week weight loss.

   Because individuals with DM type 2 are generally hyperinsulinemic, diet prescriptions for weight loss and maintenance require a lower caloric level than previously mentioned. The activity factor in kilocalories (300–400 kcal/day) can be modified in these individuals. For the type 2 DM patient, caloric restriction is of major importance. In contrast, diet for the type 1 DM patient should involve careful consistency of carbohydrate intake. Achieving this degree of dietary education generally requires several sessions with a dietitian/nutrition specialist. Dietary principles are an ongoing exercise, and eradication of myths and misconceptions is a major task. Unfortunately, many patients still perceive that "sugar-free" implies carbohydrate-free and that "sugar-free" foods cannot affect blood glucose control. This belief fails to recognize the monomer/polymer concept and the fact that most carbohydrates are ultimately digested into glucose. In addition to maintaining carbohydrate consistency, patients must learn carbohydrate augmentation for physical activity in the absence of insulin reduction. Patients also need instruction on carbohydrate strategies for dealing with intercurrent illness when the usual complex carbohydrate may be substituted with simple carbohydrate. Although it has long been said that diet is the cornerstone of DM management,[26] effective DM dietary education is still problematic owing to time constraints and reimbursement problems.

Insulin-treated patients must be aware of the many facets of insulin therapy. Accurate drawing-up and mixing of insulin is an assumption that is often not founded in reality. Site selection, consistency, and rotation are crucial. Insulin absorption is most rapid from the upper abdomen; the arms, legs, and buttocks, respectively, are next. We find that administering the premeal insulin in the abdomen optimizes postmeal control (assuming the use of lispro, insulin aspart, or regular insulin). In contrast, the buttocks, as the slowest absorption site, is not a good choice for premeal injections. However, the lower buttocks is an ideal site for bedtime injections of intermediate-acting insulin [neutral protamine Hagedorn (NPH)/lente] to minimize nocturnal hypoglycemia. Haphazard site selection and rotation can lead to erratic glycemic control. Because of the variability in absorption among sites, we suggest site consistency—using the same anatomic site at the same time of day (all breakfast injections in the abdomen, all dinner injections in the arms, all bedtime injections in the lower buttocks). Broad rotation within the sites is important to eliminate local lipohypertrophy.[27] The fast-acting insulin analogues, lispro with its peak action 1 hour postinjection and the new insulin aspart with its peak action 30 to 90 minutes postinjection, significantly improve postprandial glycemic control. This facilitates insulin injection timing as it is injected 0 to 10 minutes premeal. In contrast, regular insulin requires premeal timing of insulin injections (generally 30 minutes) to optimize postprandial glycemic control, as its peak effect is 3 to 4 hours after injection. Patients need a comprehensive perspective on insulin adjustments[28] for hyperglycemia, altered physical activity, illness management, travel, and alcohol consumption.

Patients need education on the pathophysiology, prevention, and treatment of microvascular complications. Education on macrovascular risk factors and their modification for prevention of cardiovascular, cerebrovascular, and peripheral vascular disease is also critical. Patients can have a considerable impact on decreasing foot problems and amputations with simple attention to hygiene (avoidance of foot soaks), daily foot inspection, and the use of appropriate footwear. These measures can greatly reduce the incidence of trauma, sepsis, and ultimately amputations.[29]

Diabetic Complications

Complications of DM include those that are specific to DM and those that are nonspecific but are accelerated by the presence of DM. The microvascular complications of DM are diabetes specific—the triad of retinopathy, neuropathy, and nephropathy. Macrovascular disease—atherosclerosis—a common complication in patients with DM, is not specific to DM but is greatly accelerated by its presence. A major misconception among patients and even physicians is that the complications of DM tend to be less severe in patients with type 2 DM. Patients with type 2 DM or impaired glucose tolerance have greatly accelerated macrovascular disease and also suffer significant morbidity from microvascular complications.

Retinopathy

Retinopathy, the commonest cause of new-onset blindness during middle life, is broadly classified as nonproliferative (background) and proliferative. In addition, macular edema may be present in either category. Macular edema is characterized by a collection of intraretinal fluid in the macula, with or without lipid exudates (hard exudates). In nonproliferative retinopathy, ophthalmoscopic findings may include microaneursyms, intraretinal hemorrhages, and macular edema. In more advanced nonproliferative retinopathy, cotton wool spots reflecting retinal ischemia can be noted. In proliferative retinopathy, worsening retinal ischemia results in neovascularization, preretinal or vitreous hemorrhage and fibrous tissue proliferation. Macular edema can also occur in proliferative retinopathy. Early diagnosis and treatment with laser therapy has been shown to be vision sparing in patients with macular edema and/or proliferative retinopathy. Several studies clearly document the importance of annual examinations by an ophthalmologist for all patients.[30] Good visual acuity does not exclude significant retinal pathology; unfortunately, many patients, and health care providers alike, believe good visual acuity implies an absence of significant retinal disease.

Neuropathy

The clinical spectrum of diabetic neuropathy is outlined in Table 13.2.

Nephropathy/Hypertension

Diabetic nephropathy may first manifest as microalbuminuria, detected on a spot urine determination or by the timed overnight albumin excretion rate. The presence of microalbuminuria should alert

Table 13.2. **Classification of Diabetic Neuropathy**

Type	Signs and symptoms
Sensory peripheral polyneuropathy	Pain and dysesthesia Glove and stocking sensory loss Loss of reflexes Muscle weakness/wasting
Autonomic	Orthostatic hypotension Gastroparesis, diarrhea, atonic bladder, impotence, anhidrosis, gustatory sweating, cardiac denervation on ECG
Mononeuropathy	Cranial nerve palsy Carpal tunnel syndrome Ulnar nerve palsy
Amyotrophy	Acute anterior thigh pain Weakness of hip flexion Muscle wasting
Radiculopathy	Pain and sensory loss in a dermatomal distribution

the patient and physician to the need for stringent glycemic control; such control has been shown to decrease the progression from microalbuminuria to clinical proteinuria and attendant evolution of hypertension. Hypertension increases the rate of deterioration of renal function in patients with DM, and aggressive treatment is mandatory. The Captopril Diabetic Nephropathy Study demonstrated that treatment with the angiotensin-converting enzyme inhibitor (ACEI) captopril was associated with a 50% reduction in the risk of the combined end points of death, dialysis, and transplantation in macroproteinuric (>500 mg/24 hr) type 1 DM patients. Overall, the risk of doubling the serum creatinine was reduced by 48% in captopril-treated patients. The beneficial effects were seen in both normotensive and hypertensive patients such that captopril at a dose of 25 mg po tid is approved for use in normotensive proteinuric (>500 mg/24 hr) type 1 DM patients.[31] In light of this and other studies in both type 1 and type 2 DM patients, the use of ACEI for prevention of progression of microalbuminuria and macroalbuminuria is recommended, unless there is a contraindication. For antihypertensive therapy ACEI is the antihypertensive of choice, unless contraindicated, given the data not only in nephropathy but also in retinopathy. The recent Heart Outcomes Prevention Evaluation (HOPE) study demonstrated a reduced risk of microvascular and macrovascular events in individuals with DM treated with the ACEI ramipril.[32,33]

Given the macrovascular benefits alone, we should probably be looking for reasons not to prescribe ACEIs, rather than reasons to prescribe them. In patients intolerant of ACEIs due to cough, angiotensin receptor blockers and calcium channel blockers are good alternatives in light of data that show decreasing proteinuria with many of these agents over and above that achievable with conventional antihypertensive therapy. Additionally, beta-blockers have a favorable metabolic and side-effect profile. Avoidance of excessive dietary protein intake is also important, as excessive dietary protein may be involved in renal hypertrophy and glomerular hyperfiltration. Strict glycemic control even over a 3-week period can decrease renal size (as seen on ultrasonography) and decrease the hyperfiltration associated with amino acid infusions to levels comparable to those of normal, non-DM individuals.[34] Nationwide clinical trials with pimagedine (an inhibitor of protein glycosylation and cross-linking) in diabetic nephropathy were discontinued due to adverse events and efficacy issues. Newer generation inhibitors of glycosylation and cross-linking are under clinical development.

Patients with DM in general are salt-sensitive, having diminished ability to excrete a sodium load with an attendant rise in blood pressure; therefore, avoidance of excessive dietary sodium intake is important. Hyperinsulinemia and insulin resistance are also important in the genesis of hypertension, with insulin-resistant patients having higher circu-lating insulin levels to maintain normal glucose levels. Associated with this insulin resistance and hyperinsulinemia is the occurrence of elevated blood pressures even in nondiabetic individuals. Insulin is antinatriuretic and stimulates the sympathetic nervous system; both mechanisms may be important in the genesis of hypertension. Hypertension exacerbates retinopathy, nephropathy, and macrovascular disease and must be diagnosed early and managed aggressively. When lifestyle modifications fail to control blood pressure, the pharmacologic agent chosen should be not only efficacious but kind to the metabolic milieu. Diuretics are very useful in edematous states. Beta-blockers have an important role in the post–myocardial infarction/anginal patient and in the heart failure patient. The benefits of beta-blockade in these patients outweigh the theoretical problems of masking of hypoglycemia, delay in recovery of hypoglycemia, and the worsening of insulin resistance. ACEIs inhibitors are a good choice in the proteinuric patient; calcium channel blockers are a good choice for the angina patient. Alpha-blockers are a good choice in the patient with benign prostatic hyperplasia, however, they are generally not used as monotherapy given the data suggesting increased risk of congestive heart failure.[35] Monotherapy of hypertension is frequently unsuccessful, especially in the setting of nephropathy, such that combination therapy is frequently needed with special attention to underlying concomitant medical problems.

Macrovascular Disease

Macrovascular disease is the major cause of premature death and considerable morbidity in individuals with DM, especially those with type 2 DM. Conventional risk factors for macrovascular disease warrant special attention in DM; they include smoking, lack of physical activity, dietary fat intake, obesity, hypertension, and hyperlipidemia. Correction and control of hyperlipidemia through improved metabolic control and the use of diet or pharmacotherapy are mandatory for the DM patient. The National Cholesterol Education Program guidelines[36] are of special importance to the diabetic, as are the American Diabetes Association guidelines[1] for the treatment of hypertriglyceridemia, with pharmacotherapy now being indicated for patients with persistent elevation in triglycerides above 200 mg/dL. LDL cholesterol lowering has been demonstrated to confer greater coronary event risk reduction and mortality reduction in diabetic patients than in nondiabetic patients. DM is one of the few diseases in which women have greater morbidity and mortality than men, especially in terms of macrovascular disease, with black women bearing the greatest load.

Foot Problems

Foot problems in the diabetic are a major cause of hospitalization and amputations. They generally constitute a combination of sepsis, ischemia, and neuropathy. The presence of significant neuropathy facilitates repetitive trauma without appropriate pain and ultimately nonhealing. Additionally, neuropathy may mask manifestations of peripheral vascular disease (PVD) (e.g., claudication and rest pain) such that patients may have critical ischemia with minimal symptoms. Therefore, PVD may be difficult to diagnose on the usual clinical grounds alone. Not only may neuropathy mask clinical symptoms, the clinical signs may be somewhat confusing. Patients with less severe neuropathy may exhibit cold feet related to arteriovenous shunting, and patients with more severe neuropathy may exhibit cutaneous hyperemia related to autosympathectomy. Noninvasive vascular testing along with clinical evaluation is helpful for the diagnosis and management of PVD. Calcific medial arterial disease is common and can cause erroneously high blood pressure recordings in the extremities, confusing the assessment of the severity of PVD.

Severe ischemia with symptoms and nonhealing wounds generally requires surgical intervention. Milder symptoms and disease may respond favorably to enhanced physical activity and the use of one of the hemorheologic agents—pentoxifylline or cilostazol. Appropriate podiatric footwear and management are important to both ulcer healing and prevention of repetitive trauma.[29,37] Early PVD can readily be detected by ankle-brachial indices using a hand-held Doppler. A reduced ankle-brachial index at the posterior tibial artery in isolation has been demonstrated to be an important marker, conferring a 3.8-fold increased risk of cardiovascular death.

Achieving Glycemic Control

A recent consensus conference of the American College of Endocrinology issued revised goals for glycemic control focusing on an HbA_{1c} <6.5% and a fasting blood glucose <110 mg/dL. These new goals are in line with the International Diabetes Federation standards, which in turn are in accord with the clinical trials data.

Type 1 DM

Optimal management of type 1 DM requires an educated, motivated patient and a physiologic insulin regimen. The major challenge is physiologic insulin replacement matched to dietary carbohydrate with appropriate compensation for variables such as exercise. Physiologic insulin replacement involves intensive insulin therapy with multiple injections (three or more per day) or the use of continuous subcutaneous insulin infusion (CSII) pumps. Several regimens have been utilized to achieve glycemic control (Table 13.3). The conventional split-mix regimen combining lispro/regular and an intermediate-acting insulin in the morning before breakfast and in the evening before supper is antiquated. Its major limitation is nocturnal hypoglycemia from the pre-supper intermediate-acting insulin when stringent control of the fasting blood glucose is sought. This regimen was one of those used in the conventional group in the DCCT and was inferior at reducing the risk of complications.

Taking the split-mix regimen and then dividing the evening insulin dose—delivering lispro/regular insulin before supper and the intermediate-acting insulin at bedtime—can afford a significant reduction in the risk of nighttime hypoglycemia.[38] Most patients require 0.5 to 0.8 units/kg body weight to achieve acceptable glycemic control. There are numerous options for dosing insulin in an intensive ther-

Table 13.3. Commonly Used Physiologic Insulin Programs

Insulin program	Breakfast	Lunch	Dinner	Bed (10 P.M.–1 A.M.)
Basal-bolus humalog/regular and bid ultralente	H/R + U	H/R	H/R + U	0
Basal-bolus humalog and insulin glargine	H/R	H/R	H/R	G[a]
Tid: Humalog and NPH/lente	H/R + N/L	—	H/R	N/L[b]
Qid: Humalog/regular, ultralente and NPH/lente	H/R + U	H/R	H/R	N/L[b]
Qid: regular and NPH/lente	R	R	R	N/L[b]

[a]Do not mix insulin glargine with any other insulin in a syringe.

[b]Give injection in lower buttocks.

H = humalog; G = glargine; L = lente; N = NPH; R = regular; U = ultralente.

apy regimen. One option is to distribute two thirds of the insulin in the morning and one third of the insulin in the evening, with (1) one third of the morning dose being lispro/regular and two thirds being intermediate-acting insulin; (2) 50% of the evening insulin as lispro/regular insulin before supper; and (3) the remaining 50% as intermediate-acting insulin at bedtime (10 P.M. to 1 A.M.). These doses are modified according to individual dietary preferences and carbohydrate distribution. See Table 120.3 for other options.

Additionally, patients need algorithms to adjust their insulin for hyperglycemia, varying physical activity, and intercurrent illnesses. These individualized algorithms are based on the unit/kg insulin dose. Many episodes of severe hypoglycemia occur in the context of unplanned physical activity and dietary errors; likewise, many episodes of ketoacidosis occur during episodes of minor intercurrent illness. For physical activity, a reduction in insulin dosage of 1 to 2 units per 20 to 30 minutes of activity generally suffices pending the intensity of the activity. The other option is to augment carbohydrate intake (i.e., 15 g carbohydrate prior to every 20–30 minutes of activity). During illness it is important that patients appreciate the fact that illness is a situation of insulin resistance and that all of the routine insulin should be administered. Carbohydrate from meals and snacks may be substituted as simple carbohydrate in the form of liquids such as juices and regular ginger ale. It is important that the treatment regimen is individualized and that therapeutic options for insulin administration are discussed with each patient. In this way, patients' lifestyles can be accommodated and appropriate insulin regimens tailored.[28] For example, using a basal-bolus regimen with ultralente or insulin glargine, it is possible to delay the lunchtime injection pending the patient's time constraints; furthermore, the insulin dose can be adjusted depending on carbohydrate intake and physical activity. Inhaled quick-acting insulin is under clinical investigation. Concerns exist, however, about the vasodilatory properties of insulin and the theoretical potential for pulmonary hypotension and pulmonary edema, especially in patients with cardiac dysfunction.[39] In some individuals, a lunchtime injection is not feasible. A schoolchild or a person engaged in construction work might find it difficult to accommodate a prelunch insulin injection and might be better off with a morning intermediate-acting insulin to cover the lunchtime carbohydrate intake, with lispro/regular insulin being taken to cover the breakfast carbohydrate intake as a combined prebreakfast dose.

Severe hypoglycemia in the well-educated, adherent, motivated patient on a physiologic insulin regimen is uncommon. Most severe hypoglycemic episodes are explained on the basis of diet or exercise

Table 13.4. **Hypoglycemia Management Strategies**

Causes	Signs and symptoms	Treatment
Insulin/OHA overdose Carbohydrate omission Missed/late meal Missed/late snack	Sympathomimetic Coldness Clamminess Shaking Diaphoresis Headaches	Conscious—15 g Simple carbohydrate Juice 4 oz Regular soda 6 oz 3 B-D glucose tablets 7 Lifesavers
Uncompensated activity/ exercise	Neuroglycopenic Confusion Disorientation Loss of consciousness	Unconscious Glucagon SC[a] D_{50} 50 cc IV

[a]We do not recommend the use of gel products (e.g., Monojel) for treatment of unconscious hypoglycemia, as aspiration is a potential hazard.
OHA = oral hypoglycemic agent.

and insulin-adjustment errors.[40] The individual who is attempting to achieve true euglycemia, however, is at risk for periodic easily self-treated hypoglycemia. See Table 13.4 for management strategies. For the individual with type 1 DM who has been educated thoroughly, is on a physiologic insulin regimen with an agreed diet plan, and has algorithms for illness and physical activity, failure to attain the desired degree of glycemic control is largely related to psychosocial variables or, occasionally, altered and unpredictable insulin kinetics.

Type 2 DM

In most instances, type 2 DM is a syndrome of insulin resistance coupled with variable secretory defects, both of which can be compounded by glucotoxicity. As insulin resistance is related to genetic factors, obesity, and sedentary lifestyle, the mainstay of treatment for the type 2 DM patient is correction of insulin resistance through diet and exercise and reversal of glucotoxicity acutely through reestablishment of euglycemia. Many patients still perceive themselves to be more absolutely insulin-deficient than insulin-resistant and are willing to accept insulin therapy as a compromise in the context of failed weight loss efforts. Additionally, many patients perceive pharmacotherapy to be equivalent to a diet and exercise regimen alone, assuming the desired degree of glycemic control is achieved. Chronic nonadherence to a diet regimen with resultant failure of weight loss or progressive obesity frequently leads to mislabeling the patient as a "brittle diabetic." It is important to avoid premature and unnecessary insulin therapy in these individuals and to stress to them the importance of diet and exercise as the most physiologic approach to controlling their metabolic disorder.

Pharmacotherapy for Type 2 DM

Pharmacotherapy for type 2 DM can be directed at (1) decreasing insulin resistance and increasing insulin sensitization (metformin hydrochloride and the thiazolidinediones), (2) interference with the digestion and absorption of dietary carbohydrate (α-glucosidase inhibitors), (3) augmentation of insulin secretion and action (sulfonylureas, repaglinide, and nateglinide), and (4) insulin therapy (Table 13.5).

Decreasing Insulin Resistance/Increasing Insulin Sensitivity

Metformin hydrochloride and the thiazolidinediones work via different mechanisms. Metformin mainly inhibits the uncontrolled hepatic glucose production, while the thiazolidinediones mainly enhance skeletal muscle glucose uptake—the earliest defect in evolving type 2 DM.

Metformin (Glucophage), a true insulin sensitizer, decreases hepatic glucose production and enhances peripheral glucose utilization. It is an antihyperglycemic agent and does not stimulate insulin secretion; hence, when used as monotherapy it cannot induce hypoglycemia. Ideal candidates for treatment are overweight or obese type 2 DM patients. The potentially fatal side effect of lactic acidosis generally occurs only when metformin is used in contraindicated patients: those with renal insufficiency, liver disease, alcohol excess, or underlying hypoxic states (congestive heart failure, chronic obstructive pulmonary disease, significant asthma, acute myocardial infarction). Metformin should be discontinued the morning of (1) elective surgery that may require general anesthesia and (2) elective procedures using contrast materials (e.g., intravenous pyelogram, cardiac catheterization), and should not be restarted for 48 to 72 hours after the surgery/procedure, pending documentation of a normal serum creatinine. Adjustments in the individual's diabetes regimen will have to be made for this time period to maintain glycemic control. In the UKPDS, despite similar levels of glycemic control, the subset of obese type 2 DM patients treated with metformin had a statistically significantly lower cardiovascular event and death rate than

Table 13.5. **Oral Medications Commonly Used to Treat Type 2 DM**

Parameter	Metformin	Pioglitazone	Rosiglitazone	Sulfonylurea
Mode of action	↓ Hepatic glucose ↑ Skeletal muscle glucose utilization	↑ Skeletal muscle glucose utilization ↓ Hepatic glucose	↑ Skeletal muscle glucose utilization ↓ Hepatic glucose	↑ Insulin secretion ↓ Hepatic glucose production
Glucose effects	Fasting and postprandial	Fasting and postprandial	Fasting and postprandial	Fasting and postprandial
Hypoglycemia as monotherapy	No	No	No	Yes
Weight gain	No	Possible	Possible	Possible
Insulin levels	↓	↓	↓	↑
Side effects	GI (self-limiting symptoms of nausea, diarrhea, anorexia)	? Elevation in hepatic transaminases	? Elevation in hepatic transaminases	Potential allergic reaction if sulfa allergy Potential drug interactions (first- generation agents) SIADH
Lipid effects	↓	↑ HDL, ↓ Trigs LDL concentration unaltered	Increase in total cholesterol, LDL and HDL concentration ? Change in particle composition	↑ or ↓

(continued)

Table 13.5 (Continued).

Parameter	Metformin	Pioglitazone	Rosiglitazone	Sulfonylurea
Usual starting dose for a 70-kg man	500 mg bid with meals or XR 500 mg with the evening meal	15 mg qd	4 mg daily either single or divided dose Better results with divided dose	Varies with each agent Glyburide 2.5 mg qd Glucotrol XL 5 mg qd Glynase 3 mg qd Amaryl 2 mg qd
Maximum dose	850 mg tid with meals or XR 2000 mg with the evening meal	45 mg qd	8 mg daily as either single or divided dose Better results with divided dose	Varies with each agent Glyburide 10 mg bid Glucotrol XL 20 mg qd Glynase 6 mg bid Amaryl 8 mg qd
Contraindications	Type 1 diabetes Renal dysfunction Hepatic dysfunction History of EtOH abuse Chronic conditions associated with hypoxia (asthma, COPD, CHF) Acute conditions associated with potential for hypoxia (CHF, acute MI, surgery)	Type 1 diabetes Liver disease Class III and IV CHF	Type 1 diabetes Liver disease Class III and IV CHF	Type 1 diabetes Hepatic dysfunction

Situations associated with potential renal failure

Parameter	Repaglinide	Nateglinide	Acarbose	Miglitol
Mode of action	↑ Insulin secretion	↑ Insulin secretion	α-Glucosidase inhibition ↓ carbohydrate digestion and absorption from GI tract	α-glucosidase inhibition ↓ carbohydrate digestion and absorption from GI tract
Glucose effects	Postprandial and fasting	Postprandial	Postprandial	Postprandial
Hypoglycemia as monotherapy	Yes; less than that seen with sulfonylureas	No	No	No
Weight gain	No		No	No
Insulin levels	↑	↑	↓ or ∇®	↓ or ∇®
Side effects	Rare hypoglycemia	Very rare hypoglycemia, as effects are glucose-dependent	GI (flatulence, abdominal distention, diarrhea)	GI (flatulence, abdominal distention, diarrhea)
Lipid effects	No change	No change	↓ or ∇®	↓ or ∇®

(continued)

Table 13.5 (Continued).

Parameter	Repaglinide	Nateglinide	Acarbose	Miglitol
Starting dose for a 70-kg man	0.5 mg prior to meals	120 mg tid prior to meals	25 mg tid with first bite of each meal	25 mg tid with first bite of each meal
Maximum dose	16 mg daily in divided doses at meals/snacks	120 mg tid prior to meals	100 mg tid with first bite of each meal	100 mg tid with first bite of each meal
Contraindications	Type 1 diabetes	Type 1 diabetes	Type 1 diabetes Inflammatory bowel disease Bowel obstruction Cirrhosis Chronic conditions with maldigestion or malabsorption	Type 1 diabetes Inflammatory bowel disease Bowel obstruction Cirrhosis Chronic conditions with maldigestion and malabsorption

the other groups.[41] Thus, metformin must be modulating other aspects of the cardiodysmetabolic syndrome.

Thiazolidinediones [pioglitazone (ACTOS) and rosiglitazone (Avandia)] are antihyperglycemic insulin-sensitizing agents that bind to the peroxisome proliferator-activated receptor (PPAR) and amplify the insulin signal. In addition to glucose lowering properties, they have purported beneficial effects on the other components of the cardiodysmetabolic syndrome. These agents may also assist in preservation of β-cell function via reduction in lipid deposition within the islets of Langerhans—a concept called lipotoxicity, a finding documented in animals. These agents can be safely used in patients with renal insufficiency without the need for dosage adjustment. A contraindication to their use is liver disease or elevations in hepatic transaminases. Edema is the commonest clinical adverse effect. Although the risk of transaminase elevation is rare, monitoring should be done every 2 months for the first year, and periodically thereafter. These agents are contraindicated in patients with New York grade III or grade IV congestive heart failure. Clinically, glucose lowering is very gradual with these agents, such that individualized downward titration in insulin dosage in insulin-treated type 2 DM patients may not be needed for at least 2 weeks, and the maximum effect may not be seen for up to 12 weeks.

α-Glucosidase Inhibition

α-Glucosidase inhibition by acarbose (Precose) and miglitol (Glyset) has a primary mode of action of decreasing postprandial blood glucoses via direct interference with the digestion and absorption of dietary carbohydrate. These agents are most commonly used as adjunctive therapy rather than monotherapy. Both of these agents need to be dosed with the first bite of the meal. Increased intestinal gas formation, the most common side effect, is minimized with slow dose titration and does improve with continued administration.

Augmentation of Insulin Secretion

Sulfonylureas enhance insulin secretion and action. First-generation sulfonylureas (chlorpropamide, tolazamide, tolbutamide), although efficacious, have a higher risk of side effects, such as sustained hypoglycemia, the chlorpropamide flush (an Antabuse-like reaction), protein binding interference with certain medications, and syndrome of inappropriate diuretic hormone (SIADH) secretion. The second- and third-generation sulfonylureas are preferred owing to their increased milligram potency, shorter duration of action, and better side-effect profile.

Prior concerns about possible cardiotoxicity of sulfonylureas related to the University Group Diabetes Program (UGDP) Study have generally disappeared, given the emergence of data to support the safety of these agents from the cardiovascular prospective in the UKPDS. Glimepiride, a third-generation sulfonylurea, has theoretical benefits in terms of reduced risk of hypoglycemia, potentially lower risk of adverse cardiovascular effects, and perhaps reduced potential for secondary failure.

The insulin secretagogue in the meglitinide class, repaglinide (Prandin), is dosed prior to meals, producing an abrupt spurt of insulin secretion, designed to assist in the control of postprandial glucose levels. There is a potential, although unproven, for a reduction in weight gain so frequently seen with sulfonylureas. Theoretical potential to reduce secondary failure rates is also a purported benefit.

Nateglinide (Starlix), a phenylalanine derivative, is an insulin secretagogue, the effects of which are glucose-dependent. Nateglinide dosed prior to meals produces an abrupt spurt of insulin. However, in contrast to repaglinide, nateglinide restores early insulin secretion that is lost as β-cell function is declining prior to the development of type 2 DM. Early insulin secretion is important, shutting off hepatic glucose production in preparation for the prandial glucose rise. Weight gain is attenuated and hypoglycemia is very rare. Switching from a sulfonylurea to nateglinide can result in a slight rise in fasting glucoses; however, as postprandial glucoses are significantly improved, the HbA$_{1c}$ may be maintained or lowered. This is due to the fact that postprandial glucose contributes more to the HbA$_{1c}$ than fasting or preprandial glucoses do.

Insulin Therapy

To achieve the American Diabetes Association (ADA) goal HbA$_{1c}$, the vast majority of type 2 DM patients will require combination therapy. The concept of initiating pharmacotherapy with an insulin-sensitizing agent appears physiologically logical and, it is hoped, will assist in delaying or preventing sulfonylurea failure, frequently seen after 5 to 6 years of sulfonylurea monotherapy. Additionally, insulin sensitization will ameliorate many of the other components of the cardiodysmetabolic syndrome, thus, it is hoped, translating to reduced macrovascular disease. This hypothesis is currently being tested in several clinical trials.

Can type 2 DM be prevented? The Diabetes Prevention Program in type 2 DM is ongoing with metformin being used in the treatment group. In the HOPE trial, that nondiabetic patients at high risk to develop cardiovascular disease who were treated with ramipril 10 mg daily had a 34% risk reduction in the development of type 2 DM.[33] In the West of Scotland trial, the use of pravastatin reduced the risk of developing type 2 DM by 30%.[42] A recent Finnish lifestyle modification study demonstrated a 58% risk reduction in developing type 2 DM in patients with impaired glucose tolerance who were randomized to a program of intensive diet and exercise.[43]

Insulin therapy in type 2 DM patients is indicated in situations where patients are acutely decompensated and are more insulin-resistant due to intercurrent illnesses. Clearly, short-term insulin therapy can reestablish glycemic control acutely in many individuals. However, reevaluation of endogenous insulin production with C-peptide determinations is important. Most obese patients with type 2 DM have normal or fairly elevated C-peptide levels, assuming they are not glucotoxic from antecedent chronic hyperglycemia. The initiation of insulin therapy in a type 2 DM patient remains controversial in terms of indications and optimum insulin regimen. The dilemma revolves around the obese C-peptide–positive patient who was achieving good glycemic control in the short term with insulin. This individual often suffers progressive obesity and worsening glycemic control owing to worsening insulin resistance, thereby increasing requirements for exogenous insulin. Thus frequently insulin therapy in an obese C-peptide–positive patient fails to achieve its primary goal of sustained improved glycemic control. Additionally, perpetuation of the obese state, or indeed worsening thereof, in conjunction with progressive hyperinsulinemia raises concerns about the impact of this worsened metabolic milieu on hypertension, dyslipidemia, and the atherosclerotic process. Initiation of insulin therapy should therefore be undertaken cautiously in most patients and progress carefully monitored in terms not only of glycemic control but also of hypertension, dyslipidemia, and obesity.

Many insulin regimens have been used to treat type 2 DM, most being similar to those used in the type 1 setting. Trends have focused on the use of bedtime insulin therapy in these individuals on the grounds that it can maximally affect the dawn hepatic glucose output/disposal and peak insulin resistance, thereby achieving the best possible fasting blood glucose and minimizing glucotoxicity. Minimizing glucotoxicity facilitates daytime islet secretory function and minimizes the need for daytime insulin therapy.[44] Combination therapy with insulin-sensitizing agents and insulin seems theoretically sound, reducing the need for exogenous insulin. The data, however, support modest improvements in glycemic control and modest reduction in insulin requirements. It is the exceptional patient who is able to discontinue insulin therapy. One such regimen has been the use of a bedtime dose of intermediate-acting insulin at a dose of 0.2 units/kg of body weight coupled with daytime oral agents. An alternative to the bedtime intermediate-acting insulin is the use of insulin glargine starting at a dose of 10 units and titrating accordingly. Although hypoglycemia is relatively uncommon in type 2 DM patients owing to their fundamental insulin resistance, it can occur in those on insulin or sulfonylureas. Sulfonylureas should be used with caution in patients with hepatic or renal impairment and the elderly.

Gestational Diabetes Mellitus

Gestational DM (GDM) is an important entity in terms of maternal morbidity, fetal macrosomia, associated obstetric complications, and neonatal hypoglycemia. GDM should be sought in all patients using current screening and diagnostic guidelines (Table 13.1). Early, aggressive management can significantly improve outcome. The initial strategy for the patient with GDM is dietary control; when the goals of pregnancy are not being achieved (i.e., premeal and bedtime glucose <90 mg/dL and 1 hour postprandial glucose <120 mg/dL), insulin therapy is initiated. Given the data linking postprandial blood glucose levels to macrosomia, it is important that postprandial glucose levels are controlled adequately and that target glucose levels are achieved.[45,46] In our center the postprandial goal is most readily and predictably reached with premeal lispro insulin. To cover basal requirements we use a small dose of prebreakfast ultralente insulin and an overnight intermediate-acting insulin. As an alternative, premeal regular insulin and overnight intermediate-acting insulin can be used. Most women with GDM have reestablishment of euglycemia immediately postpartum. These individuals, however, should be counseled on the long-term risks of prior GDM for developing overt type 2 DM, which may occur in as many as 70% of these individuals.[47] Additionally, the hazards of persistent obesity, associated insulin resistance, dyslipidemia, hypertension, and potential for premature cardiovascular death must be addressed.[48]

Individuals with type 1 DM who are contemplating pregnancy should be in optimal glycemic control prior to conception to decrease the risk of congenital malformations and the incidence of maternal-fetal complications. The achievement of two consecutive HbA$_{1c}$ levels in the nondiabetic range is recommended before conception. Alternatively, CSII may be used to readily achieve these goals. Careful follow-up by a skilled management team is essential to an optimum outcome.[46] Insulin glargine has a category C rating for pregnancy and should not be used.

Contraception and DM

The use of oral contraceptives (OCs) in women with type 1 or type 2 DM has been an area of controversy,[46] with many believing that significant elevations occur in blood glucose along with an increased risk of vascular complications. In our experience the incidence of such problems is minimal given a woman who is normotensive and has an absence of vascular disease; therefore, we believe OCs can be safely used. Even for a woman in poor glycemic control, OCs are still the most effective form of contraception.

Diabetic Ketoacidosis

Diabetic ketoacidosis (DKA) is the ultimate expression of absolute insulin deficiency resulting in uncontrolled lipolysis, free fatty acid delivery to the liver, and ultimately accelerated ketone body production. Insulin deficiency at the level of the liver results in uncontrolled hepatic glucose output via gluconeogenesis and glycogenolysis. With insulin-mediated skeletal muscle glucose uptake being inhibited, hyperglycemia rapidly ensues. The attendant osmotic diuresis due to hyperglycemia results in progressive dehydration and a decreasing glomerular filtration rate. Dehydration may be compounded by gastrointestinal fluid losses (e.g., emesis from ketones or a primary gastrointestinal illness with concurrent diarrhea). Insensible fluid losses from febrile illness may further compound the dehydration.

Diagnosis of DKA is fairly characteristic in the newly presenting or established type 1 DM patient. The history of polydipsia, polyuria, weight loss, and Kussmaul's respirations are virtually pathognomonic. Physical examination is directed at assessing the level of hydration (e.g., orthostasis) and the underlying precipitating illness. Measurement of urine ketone, urine glucose, and blood glucose levels can rapidly confirm the clinical suspicion, with arterial pH, serum bicarbonate, and ketones validating the diagnosis. A thorough search for an underlying precipitating illness remains axiomatic (e.g., urosepsis, respiratory tract infection, or silent myocardial infarction). Treatment is directed at correcting (1) dehydration/hypotension;

(2) ketonemia/acidosis; (3) uncontrolled hepatic glucose output/ hyperglycemia; and (4) insulin resistance of the DKA/underlying illness. Of course specific treatment is directed to any defined underlying illnesses.

Dehydration and hypotension require urgent treatment with a 5- to 6-L deficit to be anticipated in most individuals. Initial treatment is 0.9% NaCl, with 1 to 2 L/hr being given for the first 2 hours and flow rates thereafter being titrated to the individual's clinical status. Use of a Swan-Ganz catheter is prudent in the individual with cardiac compromise. Potassium replacement at a concentration of 10 to 40 mEq/L is critical to replace the usual deficits of more than 5 mEq/kg once the patient's initial serum potassium level is known and urine output is documented. Giving 50% of the potassium as KCl and 50% as KPO_4 appears theoretically sound, but routine phosphate replacement has not been shown to alter the clinical outcome. Bicarbonate therapy is generally reserved for patients with a pH of less than 7.0, plasma bicarbonate less than 5.0 mEq/L, severe hyperkalemia, or a deep coma. Bicarbonate is administered by slow infusion 50 to 100 mEq over 1 to 2 hours with the therapeutic end point being a pH higher than 7.1 rather than normalization of the pH. Overzealous use of bicarbonate can result in severe hypokalemia with attendant cardiac arrhythmogenicity, paradoxical central nervous system acidosis, and possible lactic acidosis due to tissue hypoxia. Intravenous insulin therapy is initiated at a dose of 0.1 U/kg/hr with rapid titration every 1 to 2 hours should a 75 to 100 mg/dL/hr decrease in glucose not be achieved. Insulin therapy at this relatively high dose is needed to combat the insulin resistance of the hormonal milieu of DKA (i.e., high levels of glucagon, cortisol, growth hormone, and catecholamines). Given that hepatic glucose output is more rapidly controlled than ketogenesis, the insulin infusion rate can be maintained by switching the intravenous infusion to dextrose 5% to 10% when blood glucose is less than 250 mg/dL. The insulin infusion is continued until the patient is ketone-free, clinically well, and able to resume oral feeding. It is of paramount importance that subcutaneous insulin be instituted promptly at the time of refeeding.

Flow sheets should be generated documenting the following:

1. Patient admission weight relative to previous weights with serial weights every 6 to 12 hours, urine ketones, and fluid balance
2. Vital signs and mental status every 1 to 2 hours
3. Bedside glucose monitoring every 1 to 2 hours
4. Urine ketones every 1 to 2 hours
5. Fluid balance

6. Blood gases and arterial pH on admission, repeating until pH is over 7.1
7. Serum potassium on admission and then every 2 to 4 hours
8. Serum ketones on admission and then every 2 to 4 hours
9. Complete blood count, serum chemistries, chest roent-genogram, electrocardiogram, and appropriate cultures on admission
10. Abnormal chemistries other than potassium repeated every 4 hours until normal.[49,50]

References

1. Clinical practice recommendations: 2001. Diabetes Care 2001;24(suppl 1):S1–S133.
2. The European patient's charter. Diabetic Med 1991;8:782–3.
3. Landin-Olsson M, Nilsson KO, Lernmark A, Sunkvist G. Islet cell antibodies and fasting C-peptide predict insulin requirement at diagnosis of diabetes mellitus. Diabetalogia 1990;33:561–8.
4. Zeigler AG, Herskowitz RD, Jackson RA, Soeldner JS, Eisenbarth GS. Predicting type I diabetes. Diabetes Care 1990;13:762–75.
5. Keller RJ, Eisenbarth GS, Jackson RA. Insulin prophylaxis in individuals at high risk of type I diabetes. N Engl J Med 1993;341:927–8.
6. Shapiro AMJ, Lakey BS, Ryan EA, et al. Islet transplantation in seven patients with type 1 diabetes mellitus using a glucocorticoid-free immunosuppressive regimen. N Engl J Med 2000;343:230–8.
7. Helmrich SP, Ragland DR, Leung RW, Paffenbarger RS. Physical activity and reduced occurrence of non-insulin-dependent diabetes mellitus. N Engl J Med 1991;325:147–52.
8. UKPDS Group. UK prospective diabetes study XI: biochemical risk factors in type 2 diabetic patients at diagnosis compared with age-matched normal subjects. Diabetic Med 1994;11:533–44.
9. DeFronzo RA. The triumvirate: B-cell, muscle, and liver: a collusion responsible for NIDDM. Diabetes 1988;37:667–87.
10. Erikkson J, Franssila-Kallunki A, Ekstrand A. Early metabolic defects in persons at increased risk for non-insulin-dependent diabetes mellitus. N Engl J Med 1989;321:337–43.
11. DeFronzo RA, Bonadonna RC, Ferrannini E. Pathogenesis of NIDDM. Diabetes Care 1992;15:318–68.
12. Clark PM, Hales CN. Measurement of insulin secretion in type 2 diabetes: problems and pitfalls. Diabetic Med 1992;9:503–12.
13. Bjornstorp P. Metabolic implications of body fat distribution. Diabetes Care 1991;14:1132–43.
14. Ferrannini E, Buzzigoli G, Bonadonna B, et al. Insulin resistance in essential hypertension. N Engl J Med 1987;317:350–7.
15. Zavaroni I, Bonora E, Pagliara M, et al. Risk factors for coronary artery disease in healthy persons with hyperinsulinemia and normal glucose tolerance. N Engl J Med 1989;320:703–6.

16. Kern TS, Engerman RL. Arrest of glomerulonephropathy in diabetic dogs by improved glycemic control. Diabetologia 1990;33:522–5.
17. Diabetes Control and Complications Trial Research Group. The effect of intensive treatment of diabetes on the development and progression of long-term complications in insulin-dependent diabetes mellitus. N Engl J Med 1993;329:977–86.
18. UKPDS Group. Intensive blood-glucose control with sulfonylureas or insulin compared with conventional treatment and risk of complications in patients with type 2 diabetes (UKPDS 33). Lancet 1998;352:837–53.
19. UKPDS Group. Association of glycaemia with macrovascular and microvascular complications of type 2 diabetes (UKPDS 35): prospective observational study. BMJ 2000;321:405–11.
20. UKPDS Group. Association of systolic blood pressure with macrovascular and microvascular complications of type 2 diabetes (UKPDS 36): prospective observational study. BMJ 2000;321:412–9.
21. National committee for clinical laboratory standards. Development of designated comparison methods for analytes in the clinical laboratory, 2nd ed., proposed guideline. NCCLS publication NRSCL6-P2. Villanova, PA: NCCLS, 1993.
22. Viberti GC. Etiology and prognostic significance of albuminuria in diabetes. Diabetes Care 1988;11:840–8.
23. Deckert T, Feldt-Rasmussen B, Borch-Johnson K, Jensen T, Kofoed-Gnevoldsen A. Albuminuria reflects widespread vascular damage: the Steno hypothesis. Diabetologia 1989;32:219–26.
24. Marshall SM. Screening for microalbuminuria: which measurement? Diabetic Med 1991;8:706–11.
25. Hamwi GL. Changing dietary concepts in therapy. In: Danowski TS, ed. Diabetes mellitus: diagnosis and treatment. New York: American Diabetes Association, 1964;73–8.
26. Wood FC, Bierman EL. Is diet the cornerstone in management of diabetes? N Engl J Med 1986;1244–7.
27. Zehrer C, Hansen R, Bantl J. Reducing blood glucose variability by use of abdominal injection sites. Diabetes Educator 1990;16:474–7.
28. Skyler JS, Skyler DL, Seigler DE, O'Sullivan M. Algorithms for adjustment of insulin dosage by patients who monitor blood glucose. Diabetes Care 1981;4:311–8.
29. Frykberg RG. Management of diabetic foot problems (Joslin Clinic). Philadelphia: Saunders, 1984.
30. Singerman LJ. Early-treatment diabetic retinopathy study: good news for diabetic patients and health care professionals [editorial]. Diabetes Care 1986;9:426–9.
31. Lewis EJ, Hunsicker LG, Bain RE, Rohde RD. The effect of angiotensin-converting enzyme inhibition on diabetic nephropathy. N Engl J Med 1993;329:1456–62.
32. The Heart Outcomes Prevention Evaluation (HOPE) Study Investigators. Effects of an angiotensin-converting enzyme inhibitor, ramipril, on cardiovascular events in high risk patients. Lancet 2000;342:145–53.
33. The Heart Outcomes Prevention Evaluation (HOPE) Study Investigators. Effects of ramipril on cardiovascular and microvascular outcomes

in people with diabetes mellitus: results of the HOPE study and MICRO-HOPE sub-study. Lancet 2000;345:253–9.

34. Tuttle KR, Bruton JL, Perusek MC, Lancaster JL, Kopp DT, DeFronzo RA. Effect of strict glycemic control on renal enlargement in insulin-dependent diabetes mellitus. N Engl J Med 1991;324:1626–32.

35. ALLHAT Collaborative Research Group. Major cardiovascular events in hypertensive patients randomized to doxazosin vs. chlorthalidone: the antihypertensive and lipid-lowering treatment to prevent heart attack trial (ALLHAT). JAMA 2000;283:1967–75.

36. Expert panel on detection, evaluation, and treatment of high blood cholesterol in adults. Executive summary of the third report of the national cholesterol education program (NCEP) expert panel on detection, evaluation, and treatment of high blood cholesterol in adults. JAMA 2001;285:2486–97.

37. Flynn MD, Tooke JE. Aetiology of diabetic foot ulceration: a role for the microcirculation? Diabetic Med 1992;9:320–9.

38. Skyler JS. Insulin treatment: therapy for diabetes mellitus and related disorders. Alexandria, VA: American Diabetes Association, 1991;127–37.

39. Chan NH, Baldeweg S, Tan TMM, Hurel SI. Inhaled insulin in type 1 diabetes. Lancet 2001;357:1979.

40. Bhatia V, Wolfsdorf JI. Severe hypoglycemia in youth with insulin-dependent diabetes mellitus: frequency and causative factors. Pediatrics 1991;88:1187–93.

41. UKPDS Group. Effect of intensive blood-glucose control with metformin on complications in overweight patients with type 2 diabetes (UKPDS 34). Lancet 1998;352(9131):854–65.

42. Freeman DJ, Norrie J, Sattar N, et al. Pravastatin and the development of diabetes mellitus: evidence for a protective treatment effect in the West of Scotland Coronary Prevention Study. Circulation 2001;103:346–7.

43. Tuomilehto J, Lindstorm J, Eirksson JG, et al. Prevention of type 2 diabetes mellitus by changes in lifestyle among subjects with impaired glucose tolerance. N Engl J Med 2001;344:1343–50.

44. Groop LC, Widèn E, Ekstrand A, et al. Morning or bedtime NPH insulin combined with sulfonylureas in treatment of NIDDM. Diabetes Care 1992;15:831–4.

45. Proceedings of the Third International Workshop-Conference on Gestational Diabetes Mellitus. Diabetes 1991;40(suppl 2):1–201.

46. Jovanovic-Peterson L, Peterson CM. Pregnancy in the diabetic woman: guidelines for a successful outcome. Endocrinol Metab Clin North Am 1992;33:433–56.

47. Kaufmann RC, Amankwah KS, Woodrum J. Development of diabetes in previous gestational diabetic [abstract]. Diabetes 1991;40:137A.

48. Kaufmann RC, Amankwah KS, Woodrum J. Serum lipids in former gestational diabetics [abstract]. Diabetes 1991;40:192A.

49. Kozak GP, Rolla AR. Diabetic comas. In: Kozak GP, ed. Clinical diabetes mellitus. Philadelphia: Saunders, 1982;109–45.

50. Siperstein MD. Diabetic ketoacidosis and hyperosmolar coma. Endocrinol Metab Clin North Am 1992;33:415–32.

14
Thyroid Disease

Michael B. Harper and
E.J. Mayeaux, Jr.

Thyroid diseases are among the most common endocrine disorders.[1] They may seriously affect patients' health and often require lifelong treatment and monitoring. This chapter reviews the most common thyroid problems, with emphasis on clinical presentation, diagnosis, treatment, and follow-up.

Screening for Thyroid Disease

In 2000, the American Thyroid Association released consensus recommendations on screening asymptomatic adults for thyroid disease.[2] Even though they note a serious lack of efficacy data, especially in men and younger women, they recommend measuring a thyroid-stimulating hormone (TSH) level in all patients at age 35 and every 5 years thereafter. These recommendations have not been generally accepted to date. The American Academy of Family Physicians, American College of Physicians, U.S. Preventative Services Task Force, and the Royal College of Physicians conclude there is not enough evidence to recommend screening in the general population.[3] Screening patients who are at higher risk for thyroid disease is recommended. Patients with atrial fibrillation or hyperlipidemia should be screened at least once. Annual screening is recommended for patients with diabetes or Down syndrome. Those taking amiodarone or lithium require periodic monitoring.[4]

Hyperthyroidism

Thyrotoxicosis results from excess thyroid hormone. The prevalence of this condition in the United States among adults over 55 years of age is 2%. Two thirds of these patients were taking thyroid hormone preparation.[1] Excluding excess hormone ingestion, approximately 90% of hyperthyroidism is caused by Graves' disease, and thyrotoxic nodules and thyroiditis account for almost all other cases.[5] Women are more commonly affected by hyperthyroidism than men, with reported ratios varying from 4:1 to 10:1.[5,6]

Health Risks

Hyperthyroidism causes or exacerbates several other health problems, with cardiovascular complications being most important. Atrial fibrillation is the most common complication, occurring in 8% to 22% of thyrotoxic patients, and these patients are at increased risk of stroke from atrial thromboembolism.[7] Cardiac failure, angina, myocardial infarction, and sudden death have been associated with thyrotoxicosis.[8] Thyroid storm causes multisystem involvement and carries a high risk of mortality (10–75%).[5] Calcium and bone metabolism are affected by thyrotoxicosis, leading to osteoporosis and an increased risk of bone fracture. Atrial fibrillation and osteoporosis may occur with even subclinical hyperthyroidism.[9] Periodic paralysis is a rare complication of thyrotoxicosis, occurring mostly in Orientals.[10]

Family Impact

As with any chronic disease, hyperthyroidism places stress on the family system. Among other symptoms, the affected family member may experience emotional lability, heat intolerance, and fatigue, all of which strain relationships within the family. Hyperthyroidism may be especially stressful prior to diagnosis, when the patient and family do not know an illness is responsible for these changes. Additional stress may result from reduced job performance or loss of income.

Clinical Presentation

Symptoms of thyrotoxicosis, arranged in order of frequency, are listed in Table 14.1, and the chief complaint can be any one of these symptoms. A directed history usually reveals up to eight symptoms, although some patients, especially in the geriatric age group, may report only a few.[5,11]

Table 14.1. **Signs and Symptoms of Thyrotoxicosis (in Order of Frequency)**

Symptoms/signs	Percent of patients
Symptoms	
Nervousness	88
Weight loss	83
Heat intolerance	75
Dyspnea	70
Palpitation	69
Increased sweating	62
Fatigue	58
Tachycardia	51
Eye complaints	49
Weakness	47
Increased appetite	45
Vomiting	44
Swelling of legs	38
Chest pain	36
History of fever	36
Nausea	28
Diarrhea	26
Frequent bowel movements	21
Abdominal pain	20
Swelling in neck	16
Anorexia	13
Constipation	12
Dysphagia	12
Hair loss	4
Signs	
Goiter	96
Skin changes (smooth, moist)	85
Tremor	79
Tachycardia (>100 bpm) (heart rate ≥80 bpm)	76 (HR >100)
Systolic murmur	76
Ocular signs (e.g., lid lag)	60
Brisk deep tendon reflexes	56
Pulse pressure ≥70 mm Hg	52
Bruit over thyroid	47
Atrial fibrillation	8
Gynecomastia	7
Splenomegaly	7

Source: Harper MB. Vomiting, nausea and abdominal pain: unrecognized symptoms of thyrotoxicosis. J Fam Pract 1989;29:382–6.

Patients often report weight loss, even with a history of increased appetite. Heat intolerance is usually described as preferring room temperatures cooler than do other family members or preferring winter to summer. Fatigue and weakness of proximal muscles can be reported as difficulty climbing stairs.

It is of note that abdominal symptoms of vomiting, nausea, and abdominal pain, although previously thought to be rare or present only preceding thyroid storm, may be relatively common.[11] Patients who present with these abdominal symptoms as their chief complaint may be at higher risk of missed diagnosis. Vomiting can occur without nausea and tends to be postprandial. Abdominal pain is usually epigastric or left upper quadrant in location, unrelated to meals, and described as sharp or cramping.[11]

Physical findings of thyrotoxicosis are listed in Table 14.1, and five or more are typically present. Goiter is the most frequent sign, but the enlargement may be only mild or difficult to appreciate, especially when it occupies a substernal location. The skin tends to be warm, moist, and velvety smooth. A fine tremor of outstretched hands is usually present, and deep tendon reflexes are often brisk with a rapid relaxation phase. Lid lag may be present with any cause of thyrotoxicosis; exophthalmos is specific to Graves' disease. Onycholysis may be present, typically of the ring fingers, causing separation of the nail from the distal nailbed and difficulty cleaning the nails (Plummer's nails).[5,10,11]

Laboratory Evaluation

Confirmation of clinical thyrotoxicosis is accomplished by measuring thyrotropin (TSH) by a highly sensitive assay and is further substantiated with measurement or estimate of free thyroxine (T_4) and sometimes free triiodothyronine (T_3). These hormones are clinically active only when they are not protein bound. A diagnostic approach to the patient with thyrotoxicosis is shown in Figure 14.1. Along with the TSH, initial tests are usually free T_4 and free T_3. Although the reliability of some methods has been questioned in the past, newer assays of free T_4 and free T_3 are more dependable.[5,12] Alternately, free T_4 can be estimated with the free thyroxine index (FTI). This value is obtained by measuring total T_4 and thyroid hormone–binding ratio (THBR, also known as T_3 resin uptake), which is an indirect measure of thyroid-binding protein. The FTI is calculated from the first two measurements. When THBR is normal, an elevated T_4 level confirms thyrotoxicosis. However, euthyroid patients may have an elevated total T_4 due to excess thyroid-binding proteins, such

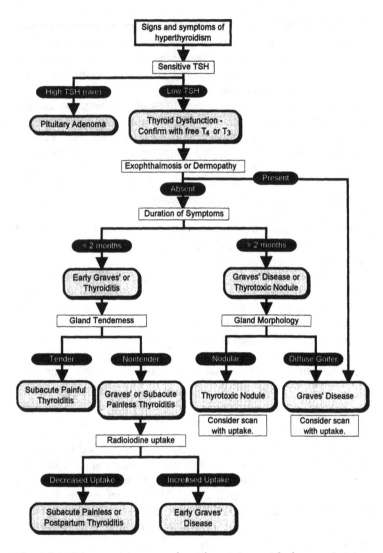

Fig. 14.1. Diagnostic approach to the patient with thyrotoxicosis.

as during pregnancy, with use of estrogens, or with some inherited disorders.

Through pituitary feedback mechanisms, TSH levels inversely follow free T_4 levels. Measurement of TSH by a highly sensitive assay in patients with hyperthyroidism yields a value far below the normal range and helps confirm the diagnosis. The sensitive TSH is especially useful in patients with concomitant illnesses or on medications that can alter T_4 and THBR values.[12] Because TSH is a more sensitive measure of thyroid status, patients may have an abnormally low TSH with a normal FTI. They are considered to have subclinical hyperthyroidism.[5,9] TSH can also be moderately low as a result of nonthyroidal illness or medications (glucocorticoids and dopamine) and is occasionally low in healthy people, particularly the elderly.[13] The TSH level in these settings is usually not less than 0.1 μU/mL. When the TSH level is less than the lower limit of a sensitive assay (undetectable), thyrotoxicosis is usually present.[5] Rarely, a TSH-secreting adenoma causes hyperthyroidism with an elevated TSH.

When TSH is low but free T_4 (or FTI) is normal, measurement of free T_3 should be obtained and, if elevated, confirms clinical thyrotoxicosis. This condition, known as T_3 toxicosis, occurs occasionally in patients with early Graves' disease or a thyrotoxic nodule.[5,10]

Nuclear medicine scans of the thyroid are useful for assessing thyroid size to determine if thyroid nodules are functioning (hot) or nonfunctioning (cold) and to measure the level of thyroid function (thyroid uptake). Of the radionuclides available for thyroid scans, iodine 123 (^{123}I) is probably optimal. Technetium may also be used for thyroid imaging, but measurement of function is less reliable, as a nonfunctioning nodule by the ^{123}I scan may demonstrate function with technetium.[5]

Graves' Disease

The disease described by Robert Graves in 1835 is the most common cause of hyperthyroidism.[10] Its etiology is an autoimmune process, closely related to chronic lymphocytic (Hashimoto's) thyroiditis. The onset of Graves' disease may follow some physical or psychological stress, and a family history of thyroid disease is often present.[5,10]

Signs and Symptoms

All the clinical manifestations of thyrotoxicosis may be present in Graves' disease, with additional specific findings of ophthalmopathy and dermopathy. A diffuse goiter occurs in most patients and may cause neck swelling or dysphagia. On palpation, the thyroid is nontender and somewhat soft. Eye problems occur in more than 50% of patients and include pressure sensation, irritation, gritty feeling, lacrimation, a change in appearance, and occasional blurred vision or diplopia. The exophthalmos occasionally causes marked eye irritation or even blindness. Dermopathy occurs in 1% to 2% of patients and causes raised, firm, nontender, intradermal nodules on the anterior surfaces of the lower legs. Clubbing of the nails (acropachy) is a rare manifestation of Graves' disease.[5,10]

Diagnosis

Graves' disease is diagnosed by confirming hyperthyroidism with thyroid function tests (FTI or free T_4), along with one or more physical findings specific to the disease. If a goiter is present without exophthalmos or dermopathy, Graves' disease may be difficult to distinguish from subacute painless thyroiditis or postpartum thyroiditis. A reliable history of chronic hyperthyroid symptoms strongly suggests Graves' disease, and an elevated thyroid uptake confirms this diagnosis when it remains in doubt.[5,10] Thyrotropin receptor (TSH-R) antibodies are present in most patients with Graves' disease but they are of limited diagnostic value. High titers of these antibodies may identify those patients who are unlikely to go into remission. Measurement of TSH-R antibodies in pregnant patients with thyrotoxicosis may be useful.[5]

Treatment

Therapy of Graves' disease is directed toward controlling the effects of excess thyroid hormone and reducing the production of additional hormone.[13] Beta-blockers are especially effective in controlling the tachycardia, tremor, and other symptoms related to excess hormone. Propranolol is begun at 20 to 40 mg two to four times daily and increased every few days until the heart rate is within the normal range.[10] When beta-blockers are contraindicated, diltiazem or clonidine may be effective.[14,15] Controlling hormone production may be accomplished with antithyroid medications, radioiodine ablation, or surgery. Choice of treatment is influenced by the clinical presentation, the age of the patient, and the patient's ability and willingness to comply with a treatment regimen.[5,10]

Antithyroid medications available in the United States to control thyroid hormone production are methimazole or propylthiouracil. In addition to blocking production of thyroid hormone, these medications may alter the course of the disease via their immunosuppressive effects.[16] Reported remission rates vary widely and are probably higher in patients with less severe hyperthyroidism, short duration of illness, and small goiter. The duration of treatment is usually 6 months to 2 years. The remission rate can be as high as 60% if treatment is continued for 2 years. Failure to achieve remission after 2 years of treatment is an indication for alternate therapy.[5,10,16]

Initial adult dosage of methimazole is 20 to 30 mg/day divided into two doses. In patients with severe hyperthyroidism and a large goiter, the higher dose is warranted. Euthyroid status, determined clinically and with thyroid function tests (T_4 and T_3), is usually achieved within 4 to 6 weeks, and the dosage is reduced incrementally every 4 to 6 weeks to a maintenance dose of 2.5 to 10 mg/day given in a single dose. TSH is not useful for following the response to treatment, as it may remain suppressed for months after T_4 and T_3 normalize. The initial dose of propylthiouracil is usually 300 mg/day, and maintenance is 50 to 100 mg/day. Both must be divided into three doses.[5,10] Either of these drugs may cause rash, leukopenia, and (rarely) agranulocytosis. Patients should be cautioned about these side effects. Methimazole has the advantages of lower risk of agranulocytosis, a longer half-life allowing usage on a once-a-day schedule, and more rapid return to euthyroid status. Propylthiouracil may be preferable during pregnancy, lactation or thyroid storm.[5,10]

Concomitant administration of thyroxine 100 to 200 μg/day has been proposed to avoid frequent adjustments in antithyroid dosage and possibly reduce recurrence of hyperthyroidism, but data demonstrating the effectiveness of this treatment regimen are limited and have not been reproduced.[5,13,17]

Iodine 131 ablation can be used to permanently destroy thyroid tissue sufficiently to reduce hormone production to normal levels. This method has become the most commonly used initial therapy for Graves' disease in the United States.[3,10] The amount of radiation used can be calculated based on the patient's weight, gland size, and thyroid uptake. In practice, this method is not strictly used because results are not as precise as desirable.[10] A major disadvantage of this treatment is the high prevalence of hypothyroidism (>90%), which continues to increase with the passage of time.[5] Therefore, a patient's ability to comply with lifelong replacement therapy should be considered when choosing this treatment.

Controversy exists regarding the use of ^{131}I ablation in children and young adults, owing to the fear of increased risk of thyroid cancer later in life. Studies to date have not confirmed this increased risk, and use of radioiodine ablation in patients under the age of 20 is common.[5,12] Pregnancy is a contraindication to [131]I. Patients who are elderly or markedly hyperthyroid should be initially treated with antithyroid drugs because ^{131}I ablation can induce a temporary exacerbation of thyrotoxicosis or thyroid storm.[10]

Subtotal thyroidectomy is an alternate method of permanently controlling thyroid hormone production. This treatment is indicated when the goiter is large, particularly if obstructive symptoms are present.

Surgery is also indicated in children who fail a trial of antithyroid medication. The disadvantages of surgery include the cost and risk of surgical complications. Following surgery for Graves' disease, hypothyroidism has been reported in 53% of patients and recurrence of hyperthyroidism in 3.4%.[10]

Follow-up

Regardless of the treatment used, Graves' disease requires lifelong monitoring. Patients treated with antithyroid medications who go into remission must be followed for possible relapses and are at a small risk of late hypothyroidism. After treatment with ^{131}I ablation or surgery, patients require chronic periodic monitoring for development of hypothyroidism. Once hypothyroidism occurs, lifelong hormone replacement is necessary.[5,10]

Thyrotoxic Nodule

An autonomously functioning thyroid nodule may cause thyrotoxicosis with typical hyperthyroid symptoms. Physical examination reveals a thyroid nodule, and findings specific to Graves' disease are absent. The diagnosis is confirmed with elevated FTI (or free T_4), low TSH, and a hot nodule on radioiodine scan. Fine-needle aspiration is indicated if the nodule is not hot on nuclear medicine scan, as with other nontoxic nodules (Fig. 14.2).

Treatment is with ^{131}I ablation or occasionally surgery. Antithyroid medications are not usually indicated for thyrotoxic nodules. Hypothyroidism following ^{131}I ablation is less common than with Graves' disease, although a 40% long-term prevalence of hypothyroidism has been reported.[18] Indications for surgery include a thyrotoxic nodule that is very large or progressively enlarging or other signs suggestive of thyroid cancer.[5]

The nodule may persist after ablation treatment, and ongoing monitoring by physical examination is needed to identify any increase in size. Should the nodule or adjacent tissue enlarge, further evaluation for possible thyroid cancer is required. Periodic monitoring for possible hypothyroidism also is necessary.

Thyroiditis

Thyroiditis is defined as an inflammatory process involving the thyroid gland. This inflammation may cause thyrotoxicosis due to unregulated release of thyroid hormone from an injured gland. There

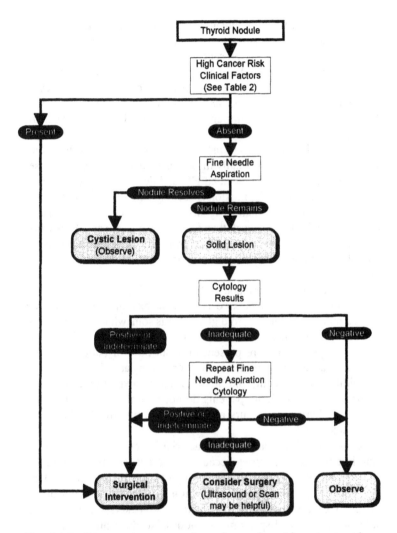

Fig. 14.2. Diagnostic approach to the euthyroid patient with a thyroid nodule.

are several types of thyroiditis, each with a different clinical picture; three are discussed below. Hashimoto's thyroiditis is discussed in the next section, and postpartum thyroiditis is discussed in the section on pregnancy. Measurement of ^{123}I thyroid uptake is useful in any patient with thyrotoxicosis and suspected thyroiditis. Elevated FTI (or free T_4) with diminished thyroid uptake confirms thyrotoxicosis due to thyroiditis.

Subacute painful (granulomatous) thyroiditis is probably caused by a viral infection and is the thyroiditis that most commonly results in thyrotoxicosis. Patients present with an exquisitely tender, firm, asymmetric nodular thyroid gland. They have symptoms of neck pain, a flulike syndrome, and symptoms of thyrotoxicosis. The erythrocyte sedimentation rate is elevated, and antithyroid antibodies are absent. These patients usually go through four phases: (1) hyperthyroidism lasting 3 to 6 weeks; (2) euthyroid status for a few weeks; (3) hypothyroidism lasting weeks to months; and (4) euthyroid state again. The clinical diagnosis is usually made during the hyperthyroid phase and is confirmed with an elevated FTI and decreased uptake on ^{123}I scans. Treatment of inflammation is accomplished with aspirin, other nonsteroidal antiinflammatory agents, or corticosteroids (prednisone 20 mg twice daily for 1 week then tapered over 2–4 weeks). Patients may require β-blocker therapy to control symptoms and tachycardia initially, but there are usually no long-term sequelae requiring treatment or monitoring.[5,19]

Subacute painless (lymphocytic) thyroiditis is an autoimmune process that may cause thyrotoxicosis. Physical examination usually reveals a mildly enlarged thyroid gland that is somewhat firm and nontender, although nearly 50% of patients have no goiter. Antibodies to thyroid peroxidase are present in about 50% of patients. These patients may go through the same four phases as subacute painful thyroiditis, but the euthyroid phase preceding hypothyroidism may be brief or absent. Some patients do not return to euthyroid status after hypothyroidism occurs and require chronic thyroid hormone replacement.[5,19]

Acute thyroiditis, caused by a bacterial infection, is a rare condition in developed countries because of the availability of antibiotic therapy. Patients present with acute thyrotoxicosis, fever, and a tender, enlarged thyroid gland. Treatment is directed toward controlling effects of excess thyroid hormone with beta-blockers and treating the infection with broad-spectrum antibiotics. Needle aspiration for culture is indicated, and abscess drainage may be necessary.[5,19]

Hypothyroidism

A deficiency of thyroid hormone can be caused by several conditions, all of which can produce the same clinical picture of hypothyroidism. The most common causes of hypothyroidism are autoimmune thyroid diseases, including Hashimoto's thyroiditis, and previous treatment for Graves' disease. Other thyroiditis, congenital hypothyroidism, and central hypothyroidism are uncommon causes.

Approximately 1% to 2% of the general population have spontaneous hypothyroidism: 1.9% of the female population, and 0.1% of the male population.[6] Hypothyroidism is more common with advancing age, affecting 6.9% to 7.3% of patients age 55 or over.[1,6] Women are affected 10 times more frequently than men. Congenital hypothyroidism occurs in 1/3000 to 1/4000 live births in the United States.[20]

Health Risks

Severe hypothyroidism may lead to coma and death if untreated. Hypothyroidism can cause bradycardia, hearing impairment, carpal tunnel syndrome, and hypercholesterolemia with increased risk of atherosclerotic heart disease. Dementia, depression, and suicide can be a sequela of hypothyroidism. Hashimoto's thyroiditis may be associated with primary thyroid lymphoma.[19] Elderly patients are at increased risk because concomitant illnesses are common and because the symptoms of hypothyroidism may remain unrecognized.[1]

Family Issues

The depression often associated with hypothyroidism has a devastating effect on the family. Withdrawal, vegetative disturbances, apathy, and loss of motivation can affect the entire family unit. This situation is especially a problem when the diagnosis is delayed.

Clinical Presentation

Symptoms of hypothyroidism include generalized weakness, fatigue, memory loss or slowed thinking, intolerance to cold, dry skin, hair loss, hoarseness, dyspnea, anorexia, deafness, chest pain, and facial or peripheral edema. A modest weight gain of approximately 10 pounds is typical, but patients may actually lose weight early in the disease process due to anorexia.[2] Constipation is a common complaint. Depression is often the presenting symptom, so hypothyroidism must be considered during any depression workup.[21,22] Women may have heavy, prolonged menstrual periods that can lead to severe anemia.[5]

Periorbital edema, peripheral edema, and pale, thick, dry skin are often the first physical signs noted. Hyperkeratosis of the knees and elbows is also common. Diastolic hypertension may be present. Delayed relaxation phase of deep tendon reflexes is common but may be subtle. When hypothyroidism is severe, mucopolysaccharides deposit in subcutaneous tissue, causing the nonpitting edema known as myxedema. Pleural and pericardial effusions, cardiomegaly, bradycardia, and prolonged QT interval are possible cardiac manifestations.[5]

Laboratory Evaluation

Hypothyroidism is diagnosed by finding an elevated TSH and a low free T$_4$ or low serum FTI.[12]

Treatment

Oral synthetic L-thyroxine is the treatment of choice for hypothyroidism.[3,12,19,20,23] The usual starting dosage is approximately 75 μg/day, but elderly patients and patients with heart disease are started at a much lower dose (25 μg/day). The TSH is measured every 6 weeks and the dosage of thyroxin is adjusted upward by 25 μg/day until the TSH is within the normal range, indicating the patient has returned to a euthyroid state. The target dose for most patients is approximately 1.6 to 1.7 μg/kg/day. Most forms of hypothyroidism are lifelong problems and continued replacement is necessary. Once the patient is on a stable dose, the TSH level should be assayed annually to monitor appropriateness of replacement therapy.[12]

There is preliminary evidence that treatment with a combination of thyroxine and triiodothyronine (12.5 μg/day) may improve mood and neuropsychological functioning in patients on replacement therapy.[24] These effects must be reproduced in larger trials before specific recommendations can be made. Addition of triiodothyronine may prove useful for patients with depression or those patients currently on desiccated thyroid preparations who are resistant to switching to thyroxine alone.

Subclinical Hypothyroidism

Subclinical hypothyroidism is defined as the presence of a high TSH with a free T$_4$ (or FTI) in the normal range. Some authors feel these patients are functionally hypothyroid relative to their own bodily requirements.[12,22,25] There is still some debate about whether to treat subclinical hypothyroidism. Patients often feel better with therapy, and treatment is usually indicated, especially if antithyroid antibodies are present.[3,4] Asymptomatic patients who have mild TSH elevation (<10 μU/mL), negative antithyroid antibodies, and no goiter may be followed without replacement.[3,5,19] Since subclinical hypothyroidism may be associated with reversible hypercholesterolemia,[26] depression,[21] and atherosclerosis,[27] treatment is warranted for patients with these conditions.

Hashimoto's Thyroiditis

Hashimoto's thyroiditis was first described in 1912 in four patients with lymphocyte infiltration, fibrosis, and follicular cell degeneration. It causes most cases of adult-onset hypothyroidism.[6,19] The etiology of the disease is autoimmune, with antibodies to thyroid peroxidase (antimicrosomal antibodies) and thyroglobulin usually present.[19,23] Like most autoimmune diseases, there is a genetic predisposition. It is most common in women (8:1) and is usually diagnosed between the ages of 30 and 50. Its incidence is increasing in developing countries.[19]

Signs and Symptoms

Patients usually present with a painless, diffuse, firm goiter. Patients may complain of tenderness or fullness of the anterior neck. Dysphagia and hoarseness are occasionally present. Although hyperthyroidism is found in up to 5% of patients during the acute stages of the disease, hypothyroidism with its various signs and symptoms is more common.[19] The presence of pain suggests the development of a primary B-cell lymphoma, a cancer associated with chronic autoimmune thyroiditis.[5]

Diagnosis

The diagnosis is suspected in patients with a characteristic goiter and is confirmed in 90% of cases by finding antibodies to thyroid peroxidase. Antithyroglobulin antibodies are also present in up to 70% of patients, but they are rarely present alone. Therefore, this latter assay is not usually necessary for diagnosis.[25] FTI (or free T_4) and the TSH level should be obtained to determine thyroid function.[19,23] If the goiter is very large, lobulated, or painful, fine-needle aspiration or biopsy may be indicated.[5]

Treatment

Treatment of hypothyroidism is described above and requires lifelong replacement. Thyrotoxicosis usually does not occur with this type of thyroiditis, and if present is of short duration requiring only symptomatic treatment. Graves' disease may precede or follow this illness and require additional treatment.

Congenital Hypothyroidism

Thyroid dysgenesis is the cause of congenital hypothyroidism in 80% of patients, and various problems with thyroid hormone production and regulation account for the rest. Severe growth and mental retardation (cretinism) can occur, but these sequelae are avoided if replacement therapy is started within the first 3 months of life. Undiagnosed congenital hypothyroidism has become rare in industrialized countries owing to neonatal screening. Transient perinatal hypothyroidism may result when mothers are given iodine or iodine-containing contrast agents.[20]

Euthyroid Sick Syndrome

Many severely ill patients have a low T_3 level or T_3 and T_4 levels below normal range. Free T_4 is usually normal if measured by a reliable, sensitive assay, and TSH is also usually normal. This so-called euthyroid sick syndrome is not indicative of true tissue hypothyroidism, and replacement is unnecessary unless the TSH level becomes markedly elevated (>20 μU/mL).[28]

Thyroid Nodules and Thyroid Cancer

Benign thyroid nodules are frequently encountered in primary care. They are estimated to occur in 4% to 8% of the adult population. In contrast, clinically significant thyroid cancer is infrequent, comprising only 1% of all malignancies and ranking 35th among causes of cancer death. Clinically insignificant thyroid cancers are more common, with American autopsy studies revealing a prevalence of 6% to 13%.[29]

Health Risks and Family Issues

Providing cost-effective yet thorough management for patients with thyroid nodules represents a distinct challenge to family physicians. Although thyroid nodules carry a low risk of mortality due to thyroid cancer, patients and their families must struggle with the knowledge that a potentially malignant growth is present. The anxiety produced by this fear not only causes stress in the patient but also has major implications for the family. Therefore, the evaluation should reveal adequate information not only to satisfy the physician but to alleviate the fears of patients and their family members.

Evaluation

Table 14.2 lists the findings that indicate high and moderate risks of cancer. When two or more of these factors are found, the probability of thyroid cancer is high. Laryngoscopy to evaluate vocal cord function is indicated, especially if any hoarseness or voice change

Table 14.2. **Clinical Factors Suggesting Malignancy in Thyroid Nodules**

High probability
  Rapid growth of nodule
  Vocal cord paralysis
  Fixation to adjacent tissue
  Enlarged regional lymph node(s)
  Very firm nodule
  Family history of multiple endocrine neoplasia type II (MEN-II) or medullary carcinoma
  Distant metastases (lungs or bones)
Moderate probability
  Age <15 years
  Age >70 years
  History of neck irradiation
  Diameter of nodule >4 cm
  Male sex and solitary nodule

has occurred. A history of neck irradiation increases the risk of both benign and malignant thyroid nodules. Multiple thyroid nodules suggest a benign process.

Laboratory Studies

Thyroid function tests and the TSH assay are useful for confirming the clinical impression of thyroid status. Thyrotoxic nodules are only rarely malignant,[5,30] although Graves' disease has been associated with an increased incidence of thyroid cancer. Measurement of antibodies to thyroid peroxidase is useful for identifying autoimmune thyroiditis when there is also diffuse enlargement of the gland. A calcitonin assay is important in patients with a family history of multiple endocrine neoplasia type II (MEN-II) or medullary carcinoma, as calcitonin is usually elevated under these conditions. Genetic testing and calcitonin elevation may identify family members with this type of thyroid cancer before clinical manifestations appear.[5,29]

Workup

The workup of a solitary nontoxic thyroid nodule is outlined in Figure 14.2. It may include nuclear medicine scans, ultrasonography, surgery, or fine-needle aspiration cytology (FNAC). The latter method has become the initial procedure of choice because it is the most accurate and most cost-effective. The FNAC technique is relatively simple and low risk,[5,29] and its sensitivity is reported to be more than 90%.[31,32] The most worrisome limitation is that a false-negative result may cause a malignancy to be missed, although the false-negative rate has been less than 10% in most studies and in one study as low as 0.7%. There is particular difficulty differentiating follicular adenoma from follicular carcinoma with FNAC, as finding evidence of invasion is required to diagnose the latter. A skilled and experienced cytopathologist is required for reliable results.

Results of FNAC are classified as positive when malignant cells are identified, negative when adequate benign glandular tissue is present, indeterminate when tissue is present and criteria for positive or negative reports are not met, and inadequate when insufficient tissue is present.[32]

Nuclear medicine scans have traditionally been part of the routine workup of thyroid nodules because a cold nodule was thought to indicate malignancy. In practice, however, scans have not proved to be as useful as expected. Because 84% of all thyroid nodules are cold on scan, most cold nodules are benign. Some thyroid cancers (1–4%) are hot on scan. Therefore nuclear medicine scans do not reliably distinguish benign from malignant nodules and so are not indicated for the routine initial workup of euthyroid patients.[5,30]

Ultrasonography can be used to determine if a thyroid nodule is solid or cystic, but this finding does not differentiate benign from malignant nodules. Studies have demonstrated that 9% to 14% of cystic nodules contain cancer compared to 10% to 20% of solid nodules being cancerous.[30] Cystic degeneration occurs in 25% of papillary carcinomas. Therefore, ultrasonography is not indicated for the routine initial workup. Ultrasonography may be used to seek the presence of other nodules, guide needle biopsy, document and follow the size of a nodule, and evaluate for metastasis.

Management

The decision regarding when to remove a thyroid nodule surgically should take into account several factors, including clinical findings, availability of FNAC with cytopathologic support, degree of anxiety of the patient and family, and ability to have reliable long-term follow-up. Reasonable guidelines are as follows: (1) Surgery is recommended for patients with one or more high-risk clinical factors or FNAC yielding positive or indeterminate results. (2) Observation is recommended for benign FNAC. Should the nodule increase in size, repeat FNAC or surgery is indicated. (3) Repeat the FNAC if the initial results are inadequate. Consider surgery if repeat FNAC is inadequate. (4) Consider surgery or repeat the FNAC for a persistent nodule after aspiration of a cyst.

Ultrasonography and nuclear medicine scans may be useful for the latter two situations when FNAC does not provide clear guidance (Fig. 14.2). Suppression of benign thyroid nodules with thyroid hormone replacement is often recommended, but the effectiveness of this treatment is questionable. If suppression is initiated, treatment for more than 12 months may be necessary to determine whether any benefit is achieved.[33] Thyroid nodules associated with Hashimoto's thyroiditis have been shown to respond to suppression.[5]

Thyroid Cancer

Four cell types of thyroid cancer are possible, each with a considerably different natural course and prognosis:

1. Papillary carcinoma accounts for 60% to 80% of all thyroid cancer. The tumor is slow-growing, and there is good long-term survival if surgical removal is performed while the cancer is still confined to the thyroid gland. Papillary carcinoma spreads by lymphatic means.
2. Follicular carcinoma accounts for 10% to 15% of all thyroid cancers. It is slightly more aggressive than the papillary variety and spreads by the hematogenous route. A subcategory of follicular carcinoma is the Hürthle cell type, which is more aggressive and more common in iodine-deficient countries.
3. Medullary carcinoma accounts for only 2% to 5% of thyroid cancers. Most of these lesions are sporadic, but some are familial; 20% are part of the MEN-II syndrome, which has an autosomal-dominant inheritance pattern. The latter can be identified early with elevated calcitonin levels and genetic testing. Screening with these tests should be performed on all family members if MEN-II or familial medullary carcinoma is diagnosed. If medullary carcinoma is not diagnosed prior to a palpable mass being present, the cure rate is less than 50%.[29,33,34]
4. Anaplastic thyroid carcinoma is the most aggressive type but accounts for only 2% to 7% of cases. It has the worst prognosis of any thyroid cancer, with a median survival time of 4 to 7 months and a 5-year survival rate of only 4%.

Surgery is the treatment of choice for all thyroid carcinoma when excision is possible. Controversy remains as to whether total or partial thyroidectomy is preferable. Near-total resection is probably the procedure of choice.[34] Radioiodine ablation is recommended for patients with known residual tumor and probably also for those at high risk of recurrence. Some patients with anaplastic thyroid cancer will respond to combined radiation and chemotherapy after thyroidecotmy.[5,24]

Thyroid Disease During Pregnancy

Both hypothyroidism and hyperthyroidism can complicate pregnancy. Thyroid-binding globulin increases during pregnancy, and so total T_3 and T_4 increase as well; hence, tests for these substances are not sufficient to diagnose or follow pregnant patients with thyroid disease.[35,36] Any use of radioactive iodine is contraindicated during pregnancy.

Hypothyroidism causes anovulation and rarely coincides with pregnancy. When hypothyroidism occurs, it is associated with gestational hypertension, premature labor, and low birth weight. Treatment consists of replacement with L-thyroxine to maintain the TSH level in the normal range on a sensitive assay.[35,36]

Hyperthyroidism during pregnancy is caused by the same etiologies as in nonpregnant patients, with Graves' disease being the most common cause. Thyrotoxicosis may lead to spontaneous abortion, stillbirth, neonatal death, and low birth weight.[35,36] Antithyroid drugs (usually propylthiouracil), propranolol, and occasionally thyroid resection may be used for treatment.[36]

Postpartum thyroiditis is a transient autoimmune thyroid dysfunction that occurs within the first postpartum year. It is probably an exacerbation of a preexisting subclinical autoimmune thyroiditis.[5,35] The true incidence is probably 5% to 10%, although it is frequently underdiagnosed.[32] The most common complaints are depression, poor memory, and impaired concentration. The clinical course consists of a hyperthyroid phase (which may be absent), followed by a hypothyroid phase and eventually a return to euthyroid status. The diagnosis is usually made with a sensitive TSH measurement. Patients with antibodies to thyroid peroxidase and thyroglobulin are at increased risk of developing this syndrome.[36] Patients who have one episode of postpartum thyroiditis are at increased risk for recurrence with future pregnancies and may develop permanent hypothyroidism.[35]

References

1. Bagchi N, Brown TR, Parish RF. Thyroid dysfunction in adults over age 55 years. Arch Intern Med 1990;150:785–7.

2. Ladenson PW, Singer PA, Ain KB, et al. American Thyroid Association guidelines for detection of thyroid dysfunction. Arch Intern Med 2000;160:1573–5.
3. Arbelle JE, Porath A. Practice guideline for the detection and management of thyroid dysfunction. A comparative review of the recommendations. Clin Endocrinol 1999;51:11–18.
4. Tunbridge WM, Vanderpump PJ. Population screening for autoimmune thyroid disease. Endocrinol Metab Clin North Am 2000;29:239–53.
5. Braverman LE, Utiger RD, eds. The thyroid: a fundamental and clinical text. 8th ed. New York: Lippincott, 2000.
6. Tunbridge WM, Evered DC, Hall R, et al. The spectrum of thyroid disease in a community: the Whickham survey. Clin Endocrinol (Oxf) 1977;7:481–93.
7. Bar-Sela S, Ehrenfeld M, Eliakim M. Arterial embolism in thyrotoxicosis with atrial fibrillation. Arch Intern Med 1981;141:1191–2.
8. Terndrup TE, Heisig DG, Garceau JP. Sudden death associated with undiagnosed Graves' disease. J Emerg Med 1990;8:553–5.
9. Sawin CT, Geller A, Wolf PA, Belanger AJ, Baker E, Bacharach P. Low serum thyrotropin concentrations as a risk factor for atrial fibrillation in older persons. N Engl J Med 1994;331:1249–52.
10. McDougall IR. Graves' disease: current concepts. Med Clin North Am 1991;75:79–95.
11. Harper MB. Vomiting, nausea and abdominal pain: unrecognized symptoms of thyrotoxicosis. J Fam Pract 1989;29:382–6.
12. Surks MI, Chopre IJ, Mariash CN, Nicoloff JT, Solomon DH. American Thyroid Association guidelines for use of laboratory tests in thyroid disorders. JAMA 1990;263:1529–32.
13. Franklyn JA. Management of hyperthyroidism. N Engl J Med 1994;330:1731–8.
14. Milner MR, Gelman KM, Phillips RA, Fuster V, Davies TF, Goldman ME. Double blind crossover trial of diltiazem versus propranolol in the management of thyrotoxic syndromes. Pharmacotherapy 1990;10:100–6.
15. Herman VS, Joffee BI, Kalk WJ, Panz V, Wing J, Seftel HC. Clinical and biochemical responses to nadolol and clonidine in hyperthyroidism. J Clin Pharmacol 1989;29:1117–20.
16. Allanic H, Fauchet J, Orgiazzi J, et al. Antithyroid drugs and Graves' disease: a prospective randomized evaluation of the efficacy of treatment duration. J Clin Endocrinol Metab 1990;8:553–5.
17. Hashizume K, Ichikawa K, Sakurai A, et al. Administration of thyroxine in treated Graves' disease. N Engl J Med 1991;324:947–53.
18. Berglund J, Christensen SB, Dymling JF, Hallengren B. The incidence of recurrence and hypothyroidism following treatment with antithyroid drugs, surgery or radioiodine in all patients with thyrotoxicosis in Malmo during the period 1970–1974. J Intern Med 1991;229:435–42.
19. Singer PA. Thyroiditis: acute, subacute, and chronic. Med Clin North Am 1991;75:61–77.
20. Gruters A. Congenital hypothyroidism. Pediatr Ann 1992;21:15–28.
21. Whybrow PC, Prange AJ, Tredway CR. Mental changes accompanying thyroid gland dysfunction. Arch Gen Psychiatry 1969;20:48–63.

22. Gold MS, Pottash AL, Extein I. Hypothyroidism and depression: evidence from complete thyroid function evaluation. JAMA 1981;245: 1919–22.

23. Rapoport B. Pathophysiology of Hashimoto's thyroiditis and hypothyroidism. Annu Rev Med 1991;42:91–6.

24. Bunevicius R, Kazanavicius G, Zalinkevicius R, Prange AJ. Effects of thyroxine as compared with thyroxine and triiodothyroxine in patients with hypothyroidism. N Engl J Med 1999;340:424–9.

25. Ladenson PW. Optimal laboratory testing for diagnosis and monitoring of thyroid nodules, goiter, and thyroid cancer. Clin Chem 1996;42: 183–7.

26. Tanis BC, Westindorp GJ, Smelt HM. Effect of thyroid substitution on hypercholesterolemia in patients with subclinical hypothyroidism: effect of levothyroxine therapy. Arch Intern Med 1990;150:2097–100.

27. Hak AE, Pols HAP, Visser TJ, Drexhage HA, Hofman A, Witteman CM. Subclinical hypothyroidism is an independent risk factor for atherosclerosis and myocardial infarction in elderly women: the Rotterdam study. Ann Intern Med 2000;132:270–8.

28. Cavalieri RR. The effects of nonthyroid disease and drugs on thyroid function tests. Med Clin North Am 1991;75:28–39.

29. Harvey HK. Diagnosis and management of the thyroid nodule. Otolaryngol Clin North Am 1990;23:303–37.

30. Cox MR, Marshal SG, Spence RA. Solitary thyroid nodule: a prospective evaluation of nuclear scanning and ultrasonography. Br J Surg 1991;78:90–3.

31. Hamming JF, Goslings BM, Steenis GJ, Claasen H, Hermans J, Velde CJ. The value of fine needle aspiration biopsy in patients with nodular thyroid disease divided into groups of suspicion of malignant neoplasms on clinical grounds. Arch Intern Med 1990;150:113–6.

32. Grant CS, Hay ID, Cough IR, McCarthy PM, Goellner JR. Long term follow-up of patients with benign fine-needle aspiration cytologic diagnoses. Surgery 1989;106:980–6.

33. Cheung PS, Lee JM, Boey JH. Thyroxine suppressive therapy of benign solitary thyroid nodules: a prospective randomized study. World J Surg 1989;13:818–22.

34. Kaplan MM. Progress in thyroid cancer. Endocrinol Metab Clin North Am 1990;19:469–77.

35. Lowe TW, Cunningham FG. Pregnancy and thyroid disease. Clin Obstet Gynecol 1991;34:72–81.

36. Bishnoi A, Sachmechi I. Thyroid disease in pregnancy. Am Fam Physician 1996;53:215–20.

15
Anemia

Daniel T. Lee and Angela W. Tang

Anemia is a reduction in blood hemoglobin (Hgb) concentration or hematocrit (Hct). Hgb values less than 14 g/dL for men and 12 g/dL for women are widely accepted to indicate anemia. However, data from large samples selected to represent the population of the United States suggests that a lower limit of 13.2 g/dL in men and 11.7 g/dL in women may be more appropriate. The lower limit of normal for children ages 1 to 2 years is 10.7 g/dL, with the cutoff rising to adult values by age 15 to 18 years. African-American references are 0.5 to 0.6 g/dL lower than for whites. There is a small decline in normal values for men but not women after age 65.[1] However, when evaluating the elderly it is advisable to use usual adult reference ranges to avoid missing important underlying disorders. In addition, it is important to evaluate results in the context of previous data. A low-normal Hgb may be significant if the value 1 week earlier was higher.

On occasion, the Hgb and Hct may not accurately reflect red cell mass. For example, patients with expanded plasma volume, as in pregnancy or congestive heart failure, may have falsely low values. Conversely, patients with plasma contraction, as in burns or dehydration, may have falsely elevated values. Finally, in the setting of acute blood loss, both red blood cells (RBCs) and plasma are lost equally, and the true degree of anemia may not be appreciated until plasma volume has time to expand.

Anemia may be categorized by cause: acute blood loss, hemolysis, or marrow underproduction. Central to this task are measurements of cell size (mean corpuscular volume, MCV) and reticulocyte count (an indicator of marrow RBC production).

Clinical Presentation

Symptoms

The degree of symptoms in anemia is highly variable, depending on the degree of anemia and the rapidity of its development. Patients may experience fatigue, weakness, and a decrease in exercise tolerance. Dizziness, headache, tinnitus, palpitations, syncope, and impaired concentration may occur. Some patients experience abdominal discomfort, nausea, and bowel irregularity as blood is shunted from the splanchnic bed. Decreased blood flow to the skin may result in cold intolerance. Patients with preexisting vascular disease are prone to exacerbations of angina, claudication, or cerebral ischemia. Those with mild or gradually developing anemias may be completely or nearly asymptomatic.

History

Historical clues assist in determining the cause of anemia. A family history of anemia or onset of anemia in childhood suggests an inherited etiology. Chronic medical conditions such as hepatic, renal, endocrine, or inflammatory disorders can lead to anemia. Malignancies and infections may cause anemia. A history of gallstones or jaundice points to hemolysis. Exposure to some medications, alcohol, and toxins (e.g., lead) can lead to anemia. Dietary intake of iron, folate, and vitamin B_{12} (cobalamin) should be obtained. Pica, especially of ice, suggests iron deficiency. Blood loss through menstruation or the gastrointestinal (GI) tract must be ascertained. Chronic diarrhea or a history of GI conditions associated with malabsorption suggests a nutritional deficiency anemia. Paresthesias of the extremities or alteration in mental status may point to vitamin B_{12} deficiency. Frequent blood donations may contribute to anemia.

Physical Examination

Tachycardia and wide pulse pressure may be present in the anemic patient. The skin and conjunctiva may demonstrate pallor. In very severe anemias, retinal hemorrhages may be seen. A systolic ejection murmur and venous hum may be heard. Jaundice may suggest hemolysis or liver disease. Glossitis can be present in vitamin B_{12} and iron deficiency. Lymphadenopathy may occur in the presence of hematologic malignancies and infections such as HIV and tuberculosis. Signs of liver disease and splenomegaly should be sought. The stool should be examined for blood. Proprioception and balance deficits may occur in vitamin B_{12} deficiency.

Table 15.1. **Classification of Anemia Based on Mean Corpuscular Volume (MCV)**

Microcytic	**Macrocytic**
Iron deficiency	Nonmegaloblastic
Thalassemia	Alcoholism
Anemia of chronic disease*	Chronic liver disease
Hemoglobin E*	Bone marrow disorders
Sideroblastic anemia*	Hypothyroidism*
Lead poisoning*	Sideroblastic anemias*
Hereditary*	Marked reticulocytosis
Myelodysplastic syndrome*	Spurious*
Severe alcoholism*	Normal variant*
Medications*	Neonatal period
Normocytic	Megaloblastic
Elevated reticulocyte count	Folate deficiency
Acute blood loss	Poor intake
Hemolysis	Malabsorption
Decreased reticulocyte count	Ethanol
Anemia of chronic disease	Medications
Chronic renal failure	Pregnancy
Chronic liver failure	Infancy
Endocrine disease	High folate requirement
Iron deficiency	B_{12} (cobalamin) deficiency
Myelodysplastic syndromes	Pernicious anemia
Aplastic anemia*	Gastric or ileal surgery*
Pure red cell aplasia*	Ileal disease*
Myelophthisic anemia*	Strict veganism*
Sideroblastic anemia*	Fish tapeworm infection*
	Bacterial overgrowth*
	Pancreatic insufficiency*
	Medications*
	Congenital disorders*
	Medications (anticonvulsants chemotherapy, zidovudine)

*Less common.

Laboratory Data

Complete Blood Count

Once a patient is determined to be anemic by Hgb and Hct, the MCV should be checked. Normal MCV for adults is 82 to 98 fL. MCV in children is lower, starting at 70 fL at 1 year of age and increasing 1 fL/year, until adult values are reached at puberty. Table 15.1 divides common causes of anemia into microcytic (<82 fL), normocytic (82–98 fL), and macrocytic (>98 fL).

The red cell distribution width (RDW) quantifies the variation in size of the RBCs. Normal RDW is less than 14.5%. An elevation of the RDW may make the MCV by itself less reliable. An example is a patient who has both iron and B_{12} deficiencies. In this case, the MCV may be normocytic, but the RDW will be elevated.[2]

Platelet and white blood cell (WBC) counts should be noted. Platelet and WBC deficiencies point to a global marrow disorder affecting all cell lines, for example aplastic anemia. Elevations suggest infection. Elevated platelet counts are often seen in iron deficiency.

Reticulocyte Count

Reticulocytes, which are newly formed RBCs, normally account for about 1% of circulating RBCs. Reticulocyte formation is increased in a normal individual who loses blood, with the degree of reticulocytosis increasing as anemia becomes more severe. Therefore, a patient's reported reticulocyte percentage should be adjusted for the degree of anemia to determine if the bone marrow response is appropriate:

Corrected Reticulocyte %
$$= \text{Reticulocyte \%} \times \text{Patient's Hct/Normal Hct.}$$

A corrected reticulocyte percentage (also known as reticulocyte index) greater than 1% indicates appropriate bone marrow response to anemia. If the value is less than 1%, causes of hypoproliferative bone marrow should be sought. Increased reticulocyte counts are present in hemolysis, acute hemorrhage, and response to treatment in anemias from other causes. An alternative to corrected reticulocyte percentage is the absolute reticulocyte count, which equals the reported reticulocyte percentage multiplied by the RBC count. The absolute reticulocyte count is normally 50,000 to 75,000/mm^3.

Peripheral Smear

Abnormalities in the peripheral smear can assist in determining the etiology of anemia (Fig. 15.1).

Other Laboratory Tests

Further laboratory testing may be warranted, depending on the MCV and reticulocyte count. Bone marrow biopsy is reserved for situations in which anemia remains unexplained or is suspected to arise from marrow dysfunction. Algorithms for evaluation of microcytic, normocytic, and macrocytic anemias are provided in Figures 15.2, 15.3, and 15.4.

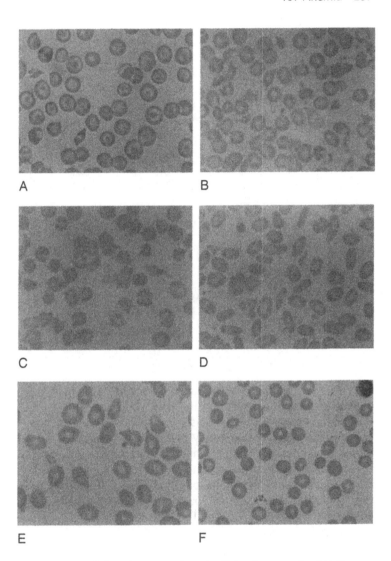

Fig. 15.1. Peripheral smear abnormalities in anemia. (A) Target cells in Hgb C, SC, E, thalassemias, and liver disease. (B) Schistocytes in microangiopathic (DIC, TTP, HUS) or traumatic hemolysis (cardiac valves). (C) Spur cells in end-stage liver disease, abetalipoproteinemia, anorexia nervosa, hypothyroidism, and splenectomy. (D) Elliptocytes in hereditary elliptocytosis. (E) Teardrop cells in myelofibrosis. (F) Spherocytes in hereditary spherocytosis and autoimmune hemolytic anemia.

(*continued*)

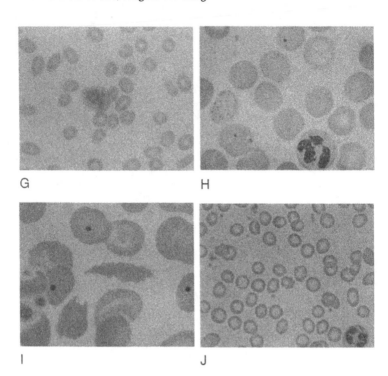

Fig. 15.1 (Continued). (G) Macroovalocytes and hypersegmented neutrophils in vitamin B_{12} and folate deficiencies. (H)
Basophilic stippling in lead poisoning, thalassemia, and sideroblastic anemia. (I) Howell-Jolly bodies in asplenia and megaloblastic anemia. (J) Hypochromia and microcytosis in iron deficiency. (DIC = disseminated intravascular coagulation; TTP =
thrombotic thrombocytopenia purpura; HUS = hemolytic ure-
mic syndrome. (Photographs courtesy of Kouichi Tanaka, MD;
Harbor-UCLA Medical Center, Torrance, CA.)

Microcytic Anemias (Fig. 15.2)

Iron Deficiency Anemia

Iron deficiency anemia (IDA) is probably the most common cause
of anemia in the U.S. The recommended dietary allowance (RDA)
for iron is 10 mg daily for men and 15 mg daily for women.[3] Daily
requirements increase during pregnancy, lactation, and adolescence.
Meats, eggs, vegetables, legumes, and cereals are principal sources

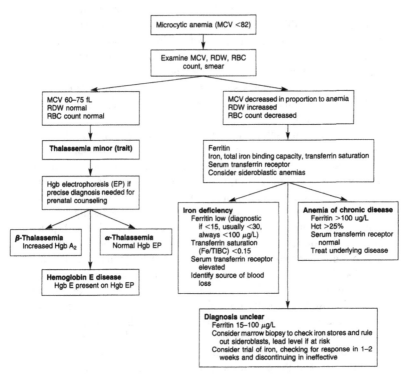

Fig. 15.2. Evaluation of microcytic anemia. MCV = mean corpuscular volume; RBC = red blood cell; RDW = red cell distribution width; TIBC = total iron-binding capacity.

of iron in the American diet, with iron from meats being much more available for absorption.

IDA is always a symptom of an underlying process that should be identified. In the U.S., IDA may be seen in infants fed primarily cow's milk because the iron content is low and the milk causes GI irritation with blood loss and malabsorption. IDA can be seen in children and adolescents whose iron needs are increased due to their rapidly growing bodies. Females lose iron in menstrual blood. Pregnancy places additional demands on a woman's iron stores as the placenta and fetus require iron and blood is lost during childbirth. In men and postmenopausal women, GI blood loss is the most likely cause of IDA. In these patients, a diligent search for occult GI bleeding is imperative when another source of bleeding is not readily appreciated. This should include upper and lower endoscopy with small bowel biopsy. Radiologic tests may substitute if endoscopy is not practical.

In over one third of patients with IDA, no source of blood loss will be found despite this evaluation.[4] In these patients, prognosis is good, with anemia resolving in more than two thirds without recurrence.[5] Further search for the source of GI blood loss is required only for persistent bleeding or transfusion dependency. IDA is also seen in decreased absorption states such as celiac disease and gastrectomy. IDA can develop in long-distance runners, probably due to blood loss from the GI tract.[6]

Physician examination may reveal glossitis and angular stomatitis. Esophageal webs, splenomegaly, and koilonychias (spoon-shaped nails) may occur rarely. The most sensitive and specific laboratory test for IDA is serum ferritin, which reflects iron stores. Ferritin below 15 μg/L is diagnostic. Since ferritin is an acute-phase reactant, however, falsely normal levels may occur with coexisting inflammatory conditions. Nonetheless, a ferritin level above 100 μg/L practically rules out IDA.[7] A decreased serum iron and increased total iron binding capacity (TIBC) are helpful but less reliable indicators of IDA. The transferrin saturation (iron/TIBC) should be less than 0.15, but this ratio may be reduced in anemia of chronic disease as well. The MCV is usually normal in early iron deficiency and typically decreases after the Hct drops. The MCV then changes in proportion to the severity of anemia. The RDW is often increased.

Occasionally, ferritin values fall in the indeterminate range of 15 to 100 μg/L and the diagnosis remains uncertain. Bone marrow biopsy is the gold standard to determine iron stores but is rarely necessary. An alternative is a several-week trial of iron replacement. Reticulocytosis should peak after 1 week, and the Hct should normalize in about a month. If no response to therapy occurs, iron should be discontinued to prevent potential iron overload. Soluble serum transferrin receptor (TfR) rises in IDA and is a promising but not widely available test that may assist diagnosis in difficult cases.[8]

Oral iron replacement is available in ferrous and ferric forms. Ferrous forms are preferred due to superior absorption and include ferrous sulfate, gluconate, and fumarate. Ferrous sulfate 325 mg tid is the cheapest and provides the needed 150 to 200 mg of elemental iron per day. However, recent studies suggest that as little as 60 mg elemental iron once or twice a week may suffice.[9] Although Hct should normalize in a few weeks, iron replacement should continue until ferritin reaches 50 μg/L or at least 4 to 6 months. Many patients experience nausea, constipation, diarrhea, or abdominal pain. To minimize these effects, iron may be started once a day and titrated up. In addition, iron may be taken with food, although this can decrease absorption by 40% to 66%.[10] Taking iron with vitamin C may help increase absorption.[11] Liquid iron preparations may be tried. Despite these measures, 10% to 20% of patients do not tolerate oral iron replacement.[12] Enteric-coated iron preparations are not well absorbed and should be avoided. Bran, eggs, milk, tea, caffeine, calcium-rich antacids, H_2-blockers, proton pump inhibitors, and tetracyclines can interfere with iron absorption and should not be taken at the same time. Also, iron supplementation can interfere with the absorption of other medications, including quinolones, tetracycline, thyroid hormone, levodopa, methyldopa, and penicillamine.

Most patients respond well to oral replacement of iron. Treatment failures may result from poor adherence, continued blood loss, interfering substances listed above, or gastrointestinal disturbances limiting absorption. In the rare case where poor absorption or severe intolerance to iron cannot be overcome, parenteral replacement may be needed. Iron dextran may be given IV or as a painful IM injection. The total dose (ml) required to replenish stores equals

$$0.0442 \times (\text{Desired Hgb} - \text{Measured Hgb})$$
$$\times \text{Weight} + (0.26 \times \text{Weight})$$

where 1 mL contains 50 mg elemental iron, and weight is lean body weight in kilograms. Adverse reactions include headache; flushing; dyspnea; nausea; vomiting; fever; hypotension; seizures; and chest, back, and abdominal pain. Urticaria and anaphylaxis can occur. A test dose (0.5 mL = 25 mg) should be given to determine whether anaphylaxis will occur. If tolerated, the remainder of the dose may be given, up to a maximum daily dose of 100 mg over 2 minutes or more. If possible, intravenous iron is preferred over intramuscular due to a lower incidence of local reactions and more consistent absorption.

Thalassemia

The thalassemias are inherited disorders of hemoglobin synthesis that are more common in people of Mediterranean, Asian, and African descent. The rare thalassemia majors cause severe anemia and are discovered early in life. Family physicians are more likely to encounter thalassemia trait (thalassemia minor) occurring in individuals heterozygous for α- or β-globin chain mutations.

Thalassemia trait should be suspected in an asymptomatic patient with mild anemia and a disproportionately low MCV (56–74 fL). The RDW is usually normal, and the RBC count is normal or increased by 10% to 20%. Iron studies are normal. Blood smear may show target cells, ovalocytes, and basophilic stippling. If a precise diagnosis is required (for prenatal counseling, for example), hemoglobin electrophoresis may be performed. In β-thalassemia trait, elevated levels of Hgb A2 and occasionally Hgb F will be seen. In α-thalassemia trait, the hemoglobin electrophoresis will be normal, and the diagnosis is made by exclusion. Treatment such as potentially harmful iron therapy is not necessary for patients with thalassemia trait.

Hemoglobin E

Hgb E has a prevalence of 5% to 30% in certain groups from Southeast Asia. The heterozygote has mild microcytosis and normal Hct. Homozygotes have marked microcytosis (MCV 60–70 Fl) and mild anemia. Target cells may be present on peripheral smear. Hgb electrophoresis reveals the presence of Hgb E, establishing the diagnosis. Hgb E is important primarily in combination with β-thalassemia; in these double heterozygotes, a severe transfusion-dependent anemia occurs.

Sideroblastic Anemia

Sideroblastic anemias are a heterogeneous group of disorders in which ringed sideroblasts are found on bone marrow staining. Sideroblastic anemia may be X linked or due to toxins or medications (lead, alcohol, isoniazid, chloramphenicol, chemotherapy). It may be related to neoplastic, endocrine, or inflammatory diseases or a part of myelodysplastic syndrome. The MCV is usually low but may range from low to high. Iron saturation and ferritin are normal to high. Marrow examination is diagnostic, and treatment is aimed at the underlying cause. In the case of lead poisoning, anemia is microcytic and basophilic stippling may be seen on peripheral smear. This diagnosis should be suspected and serum lead levels sent in high-risk groups such as children ingesting paint, soil, and dust, and adults with occupational exposure.

Normocytic Anemias (Fig. 15.3)

The absolute reticulocyte count or corrected reticulocyte percentage is important in determining the cause of a normocytic anemia.

Normocytic Anemia with Elevated Reticulocytes
Acute Blood Loss

Acute blood loss is usually obvious but can be missed in cases such as hip fractures and retroperitoneal or pulmonary hemorrhages. The

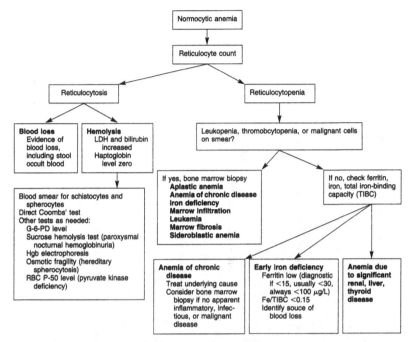

Fig. 15.3. Evaluation of normocytic anemia.

true degree of anemia may not be revealed in the Hct at first, since RBCs and plasma are lost equally. It may take several days for equilibration of blood volume and Hct to reflect fully the degree of bleeding.

Hemolysis

There are many causes of hemolytic anemia (Table 15.2). Laboratory values consistent with hemolysis include elevated serum lactate dehydrogenase (LDH) and indirect bilirubin. Haptoglobin, a plasma protein that binds and clears Hgb, drops precipitously in the presence of hemolysis. If hemolysis is suspected, the peripheral smear should be examined for schistocytes (mechanical hemolysis) and spherocytes (autoimmune hemolysis or hereditary spherocytosis), as in Figure 15.1. A direct Coombs' test will reveal an autoimmune basis for hemolysis. Further confirmatory testing may be performed as appropriate (Fig. 15.3), usually with the guidance of a hematologist. Treatment of hemolytic anemias is directed at the underlying cause and providing supportive care. Corticosteroids and splenectomy may be indicated for specific causes.

Table 15.2. **Causes of Hemolysis**

Intrinsic (defect in RBCs)	Extrinsic (defect external to RBCs)

Hemoglobinopathies
  Sickle syndromes
  Unstable hemoglobins
  Methemoglobinemia
	Immune
	  Autoimmune
	  Lymphoproliferative
	  Malignancy
	  Collagen vascular disorders
	  Drug induced (methyldopa, procainamide, quinidine, levodopa,
	    sulfas, penicillin, NSAIDs)

Membrane disorders
  Paroxysmal nocturnal hemoglobinuria
  Hereditary spherocytosis
  Elliptocytosis
  Pyropoikilocytosis
  Stomatocytosis
	Mechanical
	  Disseminated intravascular coagulation (DIC)
	  Thrombotic thrombocytopenia purpura (TTP)
	  Hemolytic uremic syndrome (HUS)
	  Prosthetic heart valves
	  Disseminated neoplasms
	  Burns
	  Malignant hypertension
	  Vasculitis
	  Severe hypophosphatemia
	  Physical activity ("march" hemoglobinuria)

Enzyme deficiencies
  Glucose-6-phosphate dehydrogenase (G-6-PD)
  Pyruvate kinase
  Glucose phosphate isomerase
  Congenital erythropoietic porphyria
	Hypersplenism
	Infections
	  Clostridium, Plasmodium, Borrelia,
	    Mycoplasma, Babesia, Haemophilus, Bartonella
	Bites
	  Snakes
	  Spiders

RBCs = red blood cells.

Normocytic Anemias with Decreased Reticulocytes

Anemia of Chronic Disease

Anemia of chronic disease (ACD), which results from chronic inflammatory disorders, infections, and malignancies, is the second most common cause of anemia after iron deficiency. It is probably the most common form of anemia in the elderly.[13] The pathogenesis of ACD is multifactorial and not fully understood. Proposed mechanisms include reduction in RBC life span, impaired utilization of iron stores, and a relative erythropoietin deficiency. Although the anemia is customarily normocytic, it can be microcytic in 30% to 50% of cases.[14] The degree of anemia is usually mild, with Hgb between 7 and 11 g/dL. The serum iron, total iron binding capacity, and transferrin saturation are usually low and not helpful in distinguishing ACD from IDA. More useful is the ferritin level, which is normal or high in ACD. Ferritin greater than 100 μg/L essentially rules out IDA, whereas levels less than 15 μg/L are diagnostic of IDA. In cases of uncertain ferritin levels (15–100 μg/L), a brief therapeutic trial of iron or a bone marrow biopsy may help with the diagnosis.

Treatment of ACD is directed toward management of the underlying disorder. Erythropoietin is effective in raising Hct in certain cases. Iron treatment will not improve the anemia, since iron stores are adequate. If the anemia is more severe than expected, one should search for a coexisting cause. For example, a patient with rheumatoid arthritis may develop concomitant IDA from GI blood loss due to chronic nonsteroidal antiinflammatory drug (NSAID) use.

Chronic Renal Failure

Anemia occurs frequently in chronic renal failure, due primarily to the kidney's inability to secrete erythropoietin. Generally, the creatinine is above 3 mg/dL. The peripheral smear is usually normal, but burr cells can be seen. The ferritin is typically increased. If a low to low-normal ferritin is noted, concomitant IDA should be entertained.

Therapy consists of ameliorating the renal failure and replacing erythropoietin. Hemodialysis may improve RBC production, but erythropoietin is the mainstay of treatment, even before dialysis is required. Complications of erythropoietin include increased blood pressure. It is important to remember that renal failure patients often have coexisting iron deficiency, and ferritin should be monitored during therapy.

Chronic Liver Disease

Chronic liver disease causes a normocytic or occasionally macrocytic anemia. Target cells can be seen on peripheral smear. Spur cells are seen in severe liver failure (Fig. 15.1). Treatment is directed at improving liver function. Alcoholics with liver disease have additional causes for anemia that are discussed under nonmegaloblastic macrocytic anemias.

Endocrine Disease

Various endocrine diseases such as hypothyroidism, hyperthyroidism, hypogonadism, hypopituitarism, hyperparathyroidism, and Addison's disease are associated with anemia. The anemia is readily corrected with treatment of the underlying endocrine problem.

Aplastic Anemia

Aplastic anemia is due to an injury or destruction of a common pluripotential stem cell resulting in pancytopenia. Bone marrow biopsy reveals severe hypoplasia and fatty infiltration. In the U.S., approximately half the cases are idiopathic. Other causes include viral infections [e.g., HIV, hepatitis, Epstein-Barr virus (EBV)], drugs and chemicals (e.g., chemotherapy, benzene, chloramphenicol), radiation, pregnancy, immune diseases (e.g., eosinophilic fasciitis, hypoimmunoglobulinemia, thymoma, thymic carcinoma, graft-versushost disease), paroxysmal nocturnal hemoglobinuria, systemic lupus erythematosus, and inherited disorders.

Treatment includes managing the underlying cause and supportive care, in conjunction with a hematologist. Judicious use of transfusions may be needed if the anemia is severe. Immunosuppressive therapy and bone marrow transplantation are indicated in certain cases.

Myelophthisic Anemia

Myelophthisic anemias result from bone marrow infiltration by invading tumor cells (hematologic malignancies or solid tumor metastases), infectious agents (tuberculosis, fungal infections), or granulomas (sarcoidosis). Less common causes include lipid storage diseases, osteopetrosis, and myelofibrosis. Treatment is directed at the underlying cause.

Red Cell Dysplasia

Pure red cell dysplasias involve a selective failure of erythropoiesis. The granulocyte and platelet counts are normal. Red cell dysplasias share many causes with aplastic and myelophthisic anemia, including malignancies, connective tissue disorders, infections, and drugs. There is an idiopathic form and a congenital form. One infection that specifically targets red cell production specifically is parvovirus B19.

This virus also causes erythema infectiosum (fifth disease), an acute polyarthropathy syndrome, and hydrops fetalis. Anemia results from parvovirus B19 infection primarily in those with chronic hemolysis (e.g., sickle cell disease), by suppressing erythropoiesis and disrupting a tenuous balance needed to keep up with RBC destruction. In this situation, anemia can be profound but is usually self-limited. Parvovirus B19 infections may become chronic in immunosuppressed individuals who cannot form antibodies to the virus. Treatment concepts for red cell aplasia are similar to aplastic anemia.

Myelodysplastic Syndromes

The myelodysplastic syndromes (MDS) are a group of clonal hematologic diseases of unknown etiology that result in the inability of bone marrow to produce adequate erythrocytes, leukocytes, platelets, or some combination of these. Patients are usually over 60 years of age and have an increased risk for leukemia. Bone marrow biopsy is diagnostic, revealing characteristic dysplastic blood precursor cells. Treatment is largely supportive.

Macrocytic Anemias (Fig. 15.4)

Macrocytic anemias may be separated into megaloblastic and non-megaloblastic types, based on peripheral smear findings (Table 15.1). A sensitive and specific sign of megaloblastic anemia is hypersegmented neutrophils, in which neutrophils contain nuclei with more than 5 lobes. A marked elevation of MCV (>120 fL) is also highly suggestive of megaloblastosis. RBCs of megaloblastic anemias, in addition to being increased in size, are often oval in shape (macroovalocytes). Most macrocytosis, however, results from non-megaloblastic causes. In a recent survey, drug therapy and alcoholism accounted for $>50\%$ of macrocytosis, whereas vitamin B_{12} and folate deficiencies accounted for only 6% of cases.[15]

Megaloblastic Anemias

Vitamin B_{12} Deficiency

Vitamin B_{12} (cobalamin) is ingested from primarily animal sources, including meats, eggs, and dairy products. U.S. RDA is 2 μg of vitamin B_{12} daily. A typical Western diet provides 5 to 30 μg/day. After ingestion, B_{12} is bound by intrinsic factor, which is produced by gastric parietal cells. Bound vitamin is absorbed in the terminal ileum. Body stores of vitamin B_{12} total 2000 to 5000 μg. Thus, B_{12} defi-

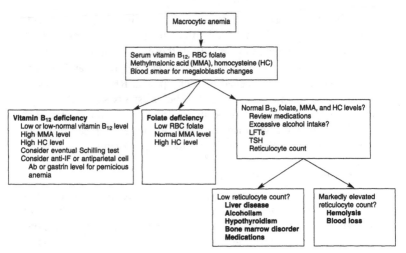

Fig. 15.4. Evaluation of macrocytic anemia. LFT = liver function test; TSH = thyroid-stimulating hormone.

ciency takes years to develop and rarely occurs from dietary insufficiency except in strict vegans. The majority of B_{12} deficiency is due to pernicious anemia, which occurs primarily in the elderly and is due to atrophy of the gastric mucosa and intrinsic factor deficiency. Other causes of B_{12} deficiency include gastric and ileal surgeries, ileal absorption problems such as Crohn's disease, sprue, and tapeworm infection.

Signs and symptoms of B_{12} deficiency include glossitis, sore mouth, and GI disturbances such as constipation, diarrhea, and indigestion. Neurologic symptoms such as paresthesias of the extremities and subacute combined degeneration (loss of lower extremity vibration and position sense) may occur. Dementia and subtle neuropsychiatric changes may be present. Importantly, anemia or macrocytosis are absent in 28% of patients with neurologic abnormalities due to B_{12} deficiency.[16]

In addition to peripheral smear changes of hypersegmented neutrophils and macroovalocytes, laboratory findings include a low B_{12} level (<200 pg/mL) and reticulocyte count. However, low-normal B_{12} levels (<350 pg/mL) are present in many patients with neurologic disease or anemia, so further workup may be indicated if the diagnosis is still suspected. Falsely low B_{12} levels may be found in folate deficiency, pregnancy, and myeloma. Elevated serum methylmalonic acid (MMA) levels are highly sensitive and essentially rule out B_{12} deficiency if normal. In one study, elevated MMA levels occurred in 98% of cases of clinically defined B_{12} deficiency. Falsely elevated levels occur in renal failure and hypovolemia, and spot urine MMA levels may be superior in this setting. Homocysteine level rises with B_{12} deficiency (96% of cases in one study) but are less specific, occurring in folate deficiency and renal disease as well.[17–19] Occasionally, a mild thrombocytopenia and leukopenia, along with an elevated LDH and indirect bilirubin from ineffective erythropoiesis, are present.

Traditionally, the Schilling test is performed to determine the etiology of B_{12} efficiency. However, B_{12} replacement effectively treats deficiencies from all causes. This test, which measures 24-hour urinary excretion of radiolabeled B_{12} given orally, distinguishes pernicious anemia from bacterial overgrowth and other absorption problems. Although the test is expensive, difficult to perform properly, and no longer available in some centers, many experts feel that it should be performed at some point during a patient's course. Alternatively, antibodies to intrinsic factor may be measured. These antibodies are highly specific for pernicious anemia but present in only about 50% of cases. Antibodies to gastric parietal cells are found in about 85% of cases of pernicious anemia but also in 3% to 10% of healthy persons.[19] Extremely elevated serum gastrin levels and low pepsinogen-1 levels also suggest pernicious anemia.

B_{12} replacement regimens vary. One common method is 1000 μg vitamin B_{12} IM daily for 1 week, then weekly for 1 month, then every 1 to 3 months for life. Hematocrit should return to normal in 2 months. Failure to normalize should trigger a search for coexisting iron deficiency, which occurs in up to one third of patients. Six months or more may be needed for neurologic improvement, and up to 80% of patients will have at least partial resolution of neurologic manifestations. An alternative to parenteral B_{12} is high-dose oral therapy. Patients with pernicious anemia can absorb 1% to 2% of oral B_{12} without the addition of intrinsic factor, so treatment with daily oral B_{12} 1000 to 2000 μg can be considered in adherent patients.[20] B_{12} maintenance can also be accomplished with an intranasal gel preparation 500 μg once weekly, although this form is more costly than parenteral and oral forms.

Folate Deficiency

Folate is found in a wide variety of unprocessed foods. Especially rich sources include green leafy vegetables, citrus fruits, liver, and certain beans and nuts. The RDA for folate is about 200 μg daily and is increased to 400 μg in pregnancy. In contrast to vitamin B_{12}, folate stores remain adequate for only 2 to 4 months, so folate deficiency anemia is often the result of inadequate dietary intake. The typical Western diet provides only 200 to 300 μg of folate daily. Persons at risk for folate deficiency include malnourished alcoholics, neglected elderly, and the homeless. Patients who are pregnant or have certain malabsorption disorders are also at risk. Impaired absorption may occur in patients taking oral contraceptives or anticonvulsants, such as phenobarbital and phenytoin. Cirrhosis can lead to deficiency through decreased storage and metabolism capabilities of the liver. Dialysis can cause loss of folate and deficiency.

The clinical findings of folate deficiency are similar to B_{12} deficiency except neurologic symptoms are generally absent. The laboratory findings are similar except that the homocysteine level is elevated (methylmalonic acid remains normal). The serum folate can rise to normal after a recent folate-rich meal, vitamin ingestion, or hemolysis, so serum folate should not be used for diagnosis. RBC folate level is felt to be more accurate, but confirmation with homocysteine levels should be obtained if the diagnosis is suspected.

Treatment is aimed at the underlying problem. Replacement is usually 1 mg orally daily. Concurrent vitamin B_{12} deficiency must be treated as well, because folate replacement can resolve hematologic abnormalities while permitting neurologic damage from cobalamin deficiency to progress.

Drugs

Certain drugs cause megaloblastic anemia. Most common causes are chemotherapy agents. Infrequent causes are phenytoin, sulfasalazine, zidovudine, trimethoprim, pyrimethamine, methotrexate, triamterine, sulfa compounds, and oral contraceptives.

Nonmegaloblastic Anemias

Alcoholism

The most common cause of nonmegaloblastic macrocytic anemia is alcoholism (also see Chapter 7). Anemia in alcoholics arises from several causes. Alcohol suppresses erythropoiesis and decreases folate absorption in patients whose diets are often poor. Alcoholics often lose blood from varices and ulcers. Anemia is worsened if liver failure occurs. Moreover, alcoholics are prone to develop sideroblastic or hemolytic anemia. They are also at increased risk for developing infections that can lead to anemia of chronic disease. Comprehensive therapy includes reduction of alcohol intake, folate supplementation, and treatment of complications.

Miscellaneous

The anemia of hypothyroidism, chronic liver disease, postsplenectomy, and primary bone marrow disorders may be macrocytic instead of normocytic. Hemolytic anemia or hemorrhage can result in macrocytosis when reticulocytes, which are larger than normal RBCs, are markedly increased. Certain drugs occasionally cause nonmegaloblastic macrocytic anemia.

Summary

Discovery of anemia should lead the physician to investigate the underlying cause of anemia. Conversely, it may be reasonable to check for anemia in patients who develop certain acute or chronic medical conditions. The history and physical examination combined with the CBC, peripheral smear, and reticulocyte count reveal the etiology in most cases. It is not uncommon to find multifactorial causes for a patient's anemia. If the type of anemia remains unclear or there is additional evidence of marrow dysfunction (pancytopenia), a bone marrow biopsy or hematology consultation may be indicated.

References

1. Dallman PR, Yip R, Johnson C. Prevalence and causes of anemia in the United States, 1976 to 1980. Am J Clin Nutr 1984;39:437–45.
2. Bessman JD, Gilmer PR, Gardner FH. Improved classification of anemias by MCV and RDW. Am J Clin Pathol 1983;80:322–6.
3. Lee GR, Herbert V. Nutritional factors in the production and function of erythrocytes. In: Lee GR, Foerster J, Lukens J, Paraskevas F, Greer JP, Rodgers GM, eds. Wintrobe's clinical hematology. Philadelphia: Lippincott Williams & Wilkins, 1999;232t.
4. Rockey DC, Cello JP. Evaluation of the gastrointestinal tract in patients with iron-deficiency anemia. N Engl J Med 1993;329:1691–5.
5. Fireman Z, Kopelman Y, Sternberg A. Editorial: endoscopic evaluation of iron deficiency anemia and follow-up in patients older than 50. J Clin Gastroenterol 1998;26(1):7–10.
6. Stewart JG, Ahlquist DA, McGill DB, Ilstrup DM, Schwartz S, Owen RA. Gastrointestinal blood loss and anemia in runners. Ann Intern Med 1984;100:843–5.
7. Guyatt GH, Oxman AD, Ali M, Willan A, McIlroy W, Patterson C. Laboratory diagnosis of iron-deficiency anemia: an overview. J Gen Intern Med 1992;7:145–53.
8. Punnonen K, Irjala K, Rajamaki A. Serum transferrin receptor and its ratio to serum ferritin in the diagnosis of iron deficiency. Blood 1997; 89(3):1052–7.

9. Gross R, Schultink W, Juliawati. Treatment of anemia with weekly iron supplementation [letter]. Lancet 1994;344:821.
10. Iron-containing products. In: drug facts and comparisons staff, eds. Drug facts and comparisons. St. Louis: Facts and comparisons, 2000;31–41.
11. Hallberg L, Brune M, Rossander-Hulthen L. Is there a physiological role of vitamin C in iron absorption? Ann NY Acad Sci 1987;498:324–32.
12. Little DR. Ambulatory management of common forms of anemia. Am Fam Physician 1999;59(6):1598–604.
13. Joosten E, Pelemans W, Hiele M, Noyen J, Verghaeghe R, Boogaerts MA. Prevalence and causes of anaemia in a geriatric hospitalized population. Gerontology 1992;38:111–17.
14. Krantz SB. Pathogenesis and treatment of the anemia of chronic disease. Am J Med Sci 1994;307:353–9.
15. Savage DG, Ogundipe A, Allen R, Stabler S, Lindenbaum J. Etiology and diagnostic evaluation of macrocytosis. Am J Med Sci 2000;319(6): 343–52.
16. Lindenbaum J, Healton EB, Savage DG, et al. Neuropsychiatric disorders caused by cobalamin deficiency in the absence of anemia or macrocytosis. N Engl J Med 1988;318(26):1720–8.
17. Savage DJ, Lindenbaum J, Stabler SP, Allen RH. Sensitivity of serum methylmalonic acid and total homocysteine determinations for diagnosing cobalamin and folate deficiencies. Am J Med 1994;96:239–46.
18. Klee GG. Cobalamin and folate evaluation: Measurement of methylmalonic acid and homocysteine vs. vitamin B_{12} and folate. Clin Chem 2000;46(8B):1277–83.
19. Snow CF. Laboratory diagnosis of vitamin B_{12} and folate deficiency. Arch Intern Med 1999;159:1289–98.
20. Elia M. Oral or parenteral therapy for B_{12} deficiency. Lancet 1998;352: 1721–2.

Index

Printed in the United States
By Bookmasters